THE PAIN OF SUICIDE:
A PHENOMENOLOGICAL APPROACH TO UNDERSTANDING 'WHY?'

(Research based on Regional Indo-Guyanese Suicidality)

Dr Jo-Ann Rowland

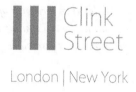

London | New York

Published by Clink Street Publishing 2019

Copyright © 2019

First edition.

ISBN: 978-1-912850-76-1 ebook: 978-1-912850-77-8

To my husband, Mr Berlon Michael Rowland

A true Servant Leader.

Every suicide is an individual tragedy whose origins can never be said to be fully understood... Every family touched by suicide is devastated by the experience and searches, as mankind has for centuries, to understand the reasons for this most unfathomable of human actions. The decision to end one's life is undeniably the ultimate most individual act.

Mayer

I empathize with all those who have died prematurely without fulfilling purpose and for those who are left with memories too heavy to hold for their loved ones gone too soon.

Dr Jo-Ann Rowland

CONTENTS

FOREWORD

When there is a discussion of any type relating to suicide within communities it's often engaged in with a whisper and a gaze of unbelieve-ableness. The whisper is due to a moment of reflection grounded in contradiction, because suicide disrupts and mainly it disrupts our assumptions about life as a meaningful endeavor. When a member of families or communities makes a definitive decision to abruptly or slowly end their lives the implications are complex and at times catastrophic for people left behind. Suicide forces us to re-evaluate life in the human ecosystem. I have experienced such complexity and dissonance within my family. The sudden blank page left behind for my family and me to stare at in our memory of my 15-year-old nephew, Nicolas.

There are volumes of available information regarding suicide, however what makes Dr Jo-Ann Rowland's work a must-read is that it dares to investigate the subject from an indispensable cultural lens, of one of the world's most endemic suicidal populations, Guyana, which is located in the northern mainland of South America. This small coastal South American country in 2012 and 2014 boasted the highest population of suicide victims in the world, and the third highest in 2016. The Census of 2012 also reveals that Guyanese religious affiliations are 63% Christian, 25% Hindu, and 7% Muslim. These statistics add to the mystery of the causes of suicide in such a densely rich ecosystem of cultural diversity and rich religious practice. What the author has courageously indulged, that other research has not, is to open an important subject and ask hard questions within a specific context. In this work the reader is introduced to suicide attempters, along with people left to live with their broken memories and pain. Dr Rowland engages the reader in matters of life and death that directly correlate with cultural and religious perspectives that are subtle, yet there are deeply embedded belief systems within the sociocultural fabric of the Indo-Guyanese community that play an important role.

The work permits anyone at any level of concern to sense the depth and range of issues that can be viewed as casual. However, as a warning to readers, be careful not to assign cause of suicidal actions with environment or mental illness. The issues are a plethora and the reasons for taking such drastic actions remain mysterious. Dr Rowland's work is an investigation that opens the door to a conversation that expands and challenges current thinking about the subject of suicide. It's not purely scientific research – in its brilliance the work delves into a spiritual or religious dimension which I feel is the missing link when it comes to academic disciplines. Her Christian perspective does not overshadow the scientific research but provides a complementary balance. Being an academician, preacher, and overall student of learning it is refreshing to read how well she has navigated between academic and spiritual disciplines to provide a unique perspective into a difficult reality. She does not utilize her religious views to compromise the research, but she recognizes that a spiritual dimension plays a significant part in the lives of people in general. No assumptions, no casting stones of judgement, she simply combines a valid research method with a Christian worldview that permits validation for her own Christian belief system and that of others.

If you are a reader who is seeking to better understand the epidemic of suicide, or an academic looking for important information to assist in your research, I think that this book will not disappoint you. What I have come to know about Dr Rowland is her commitment to serve vulnerable people and communities. This work is a tribute to her vocation to serve and engage in transformational leadership paradigms.

A note to all readers, I don't believe that suicide is a reckless act altogether performed by someone that didn't feel like life had meaning. On the contrary, I believe that when a person decides to take their own life, in many cases, they have weighed in on a part of life that many are challenged to understand. A life filled with painful shadows instead of bright and shiny days. I suggest that suicide may be the very thing that forces people to re-think, and to contemplate life as not only a meaningful gift but also to take note of a complex broken and dark reality that exist within all communities. This reality is silent and is no respecter of social class or ethnicity. It is hidden until an abrupt occurrence of suicide. In any event it causes people to pause and take note of just how mysterious life is and for a moment we must question our sense of what is normal.

Frankly speaking, when this act is attempted or accomplished, people affected by such actions are forced to visit the deeply recessed mental and emotional spaces of their own lives to validate or discard thinking that subscribes to the notion of sameness. When suicide occurs, the stark reality is that we are all not the same when it comes to survival, coveting life, and finding fulfillment in it.

I hope that you are transformed by the reading of this manuscript! I am pleased to have been asked to support such fine work.

Sincerely,

Rev. Dr Rodney D. Rogers
Strategic Consultant/Senior Pastor
Covenant International Leadership Training Institute
Christ of Calvary Covenant Church Ministries International
Covenantintlleadership.com / Christofcalvary.org

PREFACE

Suicide is the act of intentionally taking one's life. It is a global phenomenon which has long term impact on families and communities. Not only is suicide underreported but many more people attempt suicide than die from suicide.

Guyana has recorded the highest global suicide rates for 2012 and 2014. Annual suicide figures recorded in Guyana during the period 2010–2016 were consistently higher than most countries globally. Guyana's National Suicide Prevention Plan 2015–2020 highlighted that Indo-Guyanese is a high-risk group in terms of suicidality. To gain understanding of the phenomenon, I interviewed ten Indo-Guyanese, five suicide attempters and five family-member survivors of suicide completers, originating from the five Guyana regions with the highest suicidality during 2010–2016, that is, Regions 2 through 6. Interviews were digitally recorded, transcribed verbatim, and thematically analyzed using a Grounded Theory methodology. My findings were discussed within a consultation forum with key stakeholders and decision-makers. Appropriate transformational suicide intervention strategies were generated for later implementation towards the mitigation of suicides. The study found that Indo-Guyanese suicide attempts and suicides were driven by pain and hopelessness resulting from, for example, family dysfunction, alcohol and drug abuse, poor coping skills, social disconnect, leading to a devaluation of life. Family-member survivors had many unanswered questions and were hurting from painful memories, often blaming themselves for the suicide.

General awareness and targeted interventions must include government initiatives, psychosocial support such as counselling, as well as family, school, and community education and training programs, as first steps in moving towards mitigating suicides.

Reason for the Book

For over thirty years, I have been counselling individuals who have suffered diverse issues, which include mental health challenges such as depression, suicide ideation and self-harming. Additionally, for 19 years, as founder and director of a UK-based charitable organization, I have provided education, advocacy, and counselling for persons who have experienced a range of physical, mental, emotional and psychological challenges related to social isolation and exclusion as a result of homelessness and unemployment.

Around 2012, while visiting Guyana, I became aware of the high numbers of suicide being reported by the media. Guyana, with a population of less than one million people, is considered to be vividly divided along racial grounds, and driven mainly by the decisions of the two leading political parties, one mainly supported by Afro-Guyanese and the other mainly by Indo-Guyanese. I believe that this book can help to bring unity between the two races as it provides a platform for understanding and interracial sharing of experiences in a nation that is not only divided but is also hurting, as evidenced by the Indo-Guyanese suicide phenomenon. I agree with Morgan (2017), who states

> It takes ministry at the margin to rescue the man or woman living on the edge. The one called to such a ministry must himself be prepared to be marginalized... Incarnation Christians in the city must be willing to live out the Gospel of Jesus, speak like He did and be willing to serve like He did.

Serving the way Jesus served always brings healing and reconciliation, as the ultimate Counsellor, the Holy Spirit, is allowed into every dysfunctional situation.

ACKNOWLEDGEMENTS

My thanks to my husband, Michael; children, Tami, Jonathan, and David; and my grandsons, Joshua, Micah, and Malakai for being patient and understanding of the time spent away from family while generating material for this book.

My greatest thanks are to my mother, Veronica Fredericks, and my aunt, Albertha Fredericks, both deceased, who have been instrumental throughout most of my academic years, by their unstinting encouragement and motivation to me. I owe them both so much for their contributions, particularly in the early decision-making stages of my life. Thank you and I wish you were physically here at this time.

I am thankful to Professor Rodney Robinson-Rogers of Covenant Leadership Academy, who has been a great encourager. I am thankful to Dr Christopher Johnson, Pastor Kwesi Oginga and Dr. X. who were available to offer a culturally sensitive Guyanese perspective.

I am truly grateful to Pastor Iain Waddell and Social Worker Ms Lorraine Cole, who have been praying for, and encouraging me, as well as providing me with wise insights based on their personal experiences.

My special thanks go to Mrs. Karen Roberts of PAHO, all the participants and consultation meeting attendees, without whom this work would not have been possible. Thank you all for your contributions and inspiration.

PART 1
INTRODUCTION AND CONTEXT

CHAPTER 1

INTRODUCTION

"Humans are endowed with a drive for survival, yet we often do things that impede this drive. Suicide is the most extreme case."
(Nock, 2009, p. 78)

Globally, suicide is a major societal issue and is almost age-irrelevant. The World Health Organization's (WHO's) 2014 report on suicide prevention describes suicide as a global phenomenon (p. 76). According to the report, more than 800 000 people die due to suicide every year, one person every 40 seconds (p. 10). The report states that for each adult suicide death, there may have been more than 20 others attempting suicide (p. 76). The report also states that "a prior suicide attempt is the single most

> More than 800 000 people die due to suicide every year, one person every 40 seconds.

> A prior suicide attempt is the single most important risk factor for suicide in the general population.

> WHO estimates the annual global suicide rate may rise to 1.5 million by 2020.

important risk factor for suicide in the general population" (p. 10). Giddens (2007) notes that WHO estimates the annual global suicide rate may rise to 1.5 million by 2020 (p. 11).

> According to WHO (2018), over 79% of suicides occur in low- and middle-income countries.

WHO's 2014 global report on suicide ranked Guyana, in South America, as having the highest estimated suicide rate of 44.2/100,000 in 2012 (p. 86), which translated to about 200 suicide deaths in 2012. According to WHO (2018), over 79% of suicides occur in low- and middle-income countries. The World Bank (2018) indicates that Guyana is an upper middle-income economy (para. 7). Table 1 shows the Gross National Income (GNI) per capita in 2016.

Table 1

Gross National Income (GNI) per capita in 2016 Source: World Bank (2018, para. 1)

Type of Economy	GNI per capita as at 2016
Low income	$US1005 or less
Lower middle-income	Between US$1006 and US$3955
Upper middle-income	Between US$3956 and US$12,235
High income	US$12,236 or more

Guyanese suicides and attempted suicides are considered a phenomenon based on the Guyana Ministry of Public Health's (2014) report on the continued frequency, numbers, specific regional focus, and particularly because they are executed mainly by Indo-Guyanese (pp. 16–18). Suicides are described here as the fully conscious, voluntary, and intentional act of taking one's own life. The purpose of the phenomenological research presented in later chapters of this book is to uncover meaning in the phenomenon of individual acts of suicides and attempted suicides, within Indo-Guyanese communities in Guyana, South America.

Mangar (2007) described *Indo-Guyanese* as descendants of East Indian indentured labourers, who emigrated from India to Guyana, and worked mainly in the sugar and rice industries (paras. 2, 12–13). The immigrants brought with them their main religions, Hinduism and Islam, and their holy books, the Ramayana,

East Indian immigrants and their descendants were able to survive largely due to their resilience, determination, custom, tradition, and commitment to family.

4

Bhagavad Gita and Quran. "Approximately 83% of the immigrants were Hindus while 14% were Muslims. The remaining three per cent were Christians" (paras. 16-18). Mangar (2007) states "East Indian immigrants and their descendants were able to survive largely due to their resilience, determination, custom, tradition, and commitment to family" (para. 23).

Suicide prematurely separates people from families, friends, and communities. Suicide is divisive and results in much trauma. This research was not only to provide right strategies for interventions and postventions to mitigate suicide, but to give a voice to the interview participants, who have been estranged because of the stigma and loss created by suicide. Once the meaning of the suicide phenomenon is understood, there is, therefore, great potential for healing and restoration, not only for suicide attempters, but for the affected families and communities.

Problem Statement

Data collected by Guyana's Ministry of Public Health (2014) show that one of the suicide at-risk groups is the Indo-Guyanese population located along Guyana's north-eastern coast (pp. 17–18), that is, Regions 2 through 6 (Figure 1). The report shows completed suicides and attempted suicides recorded for Indo-Guyanese groups in these regions are the highest for the country. Suicides reported in Region 4, where there is a mix of Indo- and Afro-Guyanese, show it is mainly the Indo-Guyanese who have a greater tendency to commit suicide (pp. 17–18).

> Suicide prematurely separates people from families, friends, and communities. Suicide is divisive and results in much trauma.

The research sections of this book address the causes and consequences of the regional Indo-Guyanese suicide phenomenon by exploring the lived experiences of suicide attempters and family-member survivors.

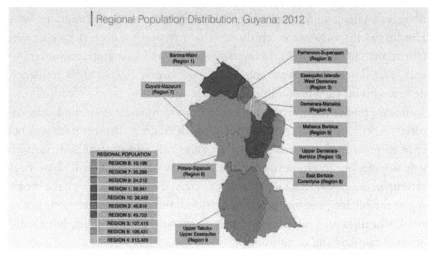

FIGURE 1. Map of Guyana, showing 10 regions. (Source Guyana Chronicles, June 30 2014). Regions 2 through 6 along the north-eastern coast experience high suicidality.

A Phenomenon

According to Guyana's Ministry of Public Health (2014), the suicide phenomenon caused Guyana to move from being the sixth highest country in the world for suicides in 2006 to having the highest estimated suicide rate in the world for the years 2012 and 2014 (pp. 8, 13).

Guyana's Bureau of Statistics (2012) census shows that Guyana has a population of 746,955 people, less than 1 million people. Guyana is split into ten regions (Figure 1 above), with Regions 2, 3, 5 and 6 being heavily populated with Indo-Guyanese. Regions 4 and 7 are mixed but Region 4 has a large number of Indo-Guyanese. Region 10 is predominantly Afro-Guyanese. Regions 1, 8 and 9 are populated mainly with Guyana's Indigenous People.

Guyana's Ministry of Public Health (2014) reported the global average suicide rate was 11.4 suicides per 100,000

East Indians (Indo-Guyanese) account for more than 80% of the suicides with most of the cases being geographically concentrated in coastal Regions 2, 3, 4, 5 and 6.

(p. 13). Generally, the suicide rate per 100,000 Guyanese is 25.6, compared with 7.3 for the Americas (p. 13). Guyana's Ministry of Public Health (2015) reported that East Indians (Indo-Guyanese) account for more than 80% of the suicides with most of the cases being geographically concentrated in coastal Regions 2, 3, 4, 5 and 6. The highest rate was found in Region 2 with 52.7 suicides for 100,000 inhabitants, followed by Region 6 with 50.8 suicides for 100,000 inhabitants (pp. 20–21). The Guyana Police Force Statistics Unit (personal communication, 2017) provided data on suicides by region during the period 2010 to 2016 and the data confirmed the high rate of regional Indo-Guyanese suicides. Figures 2 and 3 show Indo-Guyanese suicides by Region.

Indo-Guyanese Suicides by Region for the Period 2010 to 2016								
Region	2010	2011	2012	2013	2014	2015	2016	Total	Population
1	0	0	0	1	0	0	0	1	27643
2	2	0	0	7	6	5	3	23	46810
3	23	18	27	14	17	9	17	125	107785
4	26	21	20	26	19	13	19	144	311563
5	20	28	28	23	5	5	19	128	49820
6	13	4	1	13	18	23	9	81	109652
7	0	0	0	1	4	2	0	7	18375
8	0	0	0	2	1	0	0	3	11077
9	0	0	0	1	1	7	0	9	24238
10	1	0	0	2	0	0	0	3	39992
Total	85	71	76	90	71	64	67	524	746955

FIGURE 2. Data provided by Guyana Police Force in June 2017 for Indo-Guyanese Suicides by Region

Indo-Guyanese Suicides by Region 2010-2016

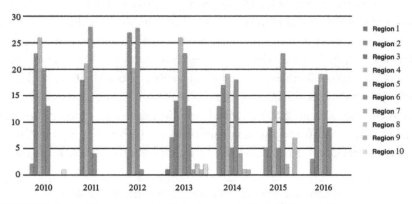

FIGURE 3. Indo-Guyanese Suicides by Region 2010-2016

Linked to the prevalence of the actual suicides, data collected by Guyana's Ministry of Public Health (2014) showed that there is an estimated ratio of 20–25 cases of suicide attempts for every suicide death and more than 50% of the suicide attempters were Indo-Guyanese (p. 18). More recent data provided by Guyana's Ministry

> An estimated ratio of 20–25 cases of suicide attempts for every suicide death and more than 50% of the suicide attempters were Indo-Guyanese.

of Public Health Statistics Unit (personal communication, 2017) showed that in 2014, a total of 266 persons attempted suicide, with 111 (42%) of that total ages 25–44 years and 98 (37%) of that total ages 15–24 years old.

Underreporting of Suicides

> Suicide rate is estimated because of the level of underreporting that exists.

The suicide rate is estimated because of the level of underreporting that exists surrounding the sensitivity of suicide data. Underreporting of suicides is not unusual because of the stigma attached to suicide and, additionally, suicide is a criminal offence in some countries, including Guyana. Tøllefsen, Hem, and Ekeberg's (2012)

8

study concluded that there was a lack of systematic assessment of the reliability of suicide statistics and as a result, there was general underreporting of suicide (p. 1). Given that underreporting is a major factor in suicide reported deaths, the figures provided by the WHO and Guyana's Ministries are also most likely to be underreported.

Past Research on Suicides in Guyana

There have been few other published studies on suicides in Guyana. An article from Edwards (2016) focused on testing traditional sociological theories, specifically Durkheim's theory of suicide and Tarde's theory of suicide, to see how they performed in assessing the high rates of suicide in Guyana (pp. 2–3). Edwards concluded that suicide in Guyana must be studied inductively to get a sense of the peculiarities of this phenomenon, in which the highest suicide rates are concentrated among one ethnic group. This ethnic group shows a high tendency to commit suicide irrespective of which geographical location they live in. Moreover, Edwards claims, that suicide seems not to have a contagion effect on other ethnic groups who live in close proximity to the Indo-Guyanese ethnic group (pp. 13–14). Gould (1990) stated that suicide contagion is a concept from the infective disease model, and assumes that a suicidal behavior may facilitate the occurrence of subsequent, similar behaviors. Contagion is a process of imitation. Theories of imitation have been postulated to explain clustering of suicides and deliberate self-harm behaviors.

A study by Henry (2015) looked at the link between suicide and suicide ideation, and the ease of access to agrochemicals by farmers. Henry (2015) investigated the social responsibility of the agrochemical industry in Guyana to manage access to, and use of, agrochemicals, with social responsibility being viewed as a mechanism for prevention (pp. 1–2).

One research on suicides in Guyana was done by Kilduff and Javers' (1978) who described how the notable American cult, Peoples Temple, came from America to set up 'Jonestown' in Guyana. More than 900 of these cult members committed suicide, about one-third of whom were children. It must be emphasized that these suicides just happened to take place in Guyana and could have occurred anywhere else globally. Although conspiracy theories, scholarly analyses, political and media versions exist on the events of

18 November 1978 in Jonestown, they only serve to generate more questions rather than bring resolution to the mass suicides which occurred. Moore's (2008) version of the Jonestown events states that:

> A charismatic, but deranged, prophet named Jim Jones founded an inter-racial church in Indianapolis in the 1950s, challenging both segregation and capitalism with a social gospel that called for racial equality and just distribution of wealth among group members... Concern about the safety of African Americans in the US led the group to establish a community in the Northwest District of Guyana... Negative publicity about the Temple in San Francisco, however, forced a rapid mass migration to the project before it could handle the influx of newcomers. As a result, housing was crowded, food was scarce, and efforts to control dissidents increased. In November 1978, California Congressman Leo Ryan visited the isolated jungle community to investigate conditions there, accompanied by journalists and relatives of Peoples Temple members. On 18 November 1978, fifteen residents of Jonestown asked to join Ryan and his party as they left. While they waited to board two small aircraft, a few young men who had followed the party from Jonestown began firing upon it, killing Ryan, three newsmen, and one defector. A dozen others were wounded, some quite seriously.
>
> Back in Jonestown, more than 900 residents gathered in the central pavilion, where Jones told them what had happened and exhorted them to drink a cyanide-laced fruit punch... Eyewitness accounts are conflicting, with some saying that people were coerced into taking poison, and others saying that people willingly drank the mixture. By the end of the day, 918 Americans in Guyana were dead: 909 in Jonestown; five on the airstrip; and four in the Temple's residence in Georgetown, the capital of Guyana.

Stephenson (2005) shared eyewitness and victim Richard Tropp's notes of the Jonestown disaster:

> It will take more than small minds, reporters' minds, to fathom these events. Something must come of this. Beyond all the circumstances surrounding the immediate event, someone can perhaps find the symbolic, the eternal in this moment—the meaning of a people, a struggle.

The causes linked to suicides are very often complex, easily involving ethical, behavioural, psychological and social factors.

Scope and Limitations

From the reports provided above for the period 2010 to 2016, the suicide phenomenon among Indo-Guyanese was evident in all the regions of Guyana in which they live. For my research, I looked at the top five regions with an estimated highest suicide rates.

Suicide and attempted suicide are seen as criminal offences in Guyana. Chapter 801: Section 96 of Guyana's 1893 Criminal Law (Offences) Act states that "Everyone who attempts to commit suicide shall be guilty of a misdemeanor and liable to imprisonment for two years" (Guyana's Ministry of Legal Affairs, 2012, p. 51). Suicide attempters and family-member survivors are aware of this law and its implications. When the law is breached, the offenders tend to shy away from public scrutiny, not only because of the legal and punitive consequences, but also from the stigma attached to suicide.

According to a *Guyana Chronicle Staff Reporter* (2010), a former Minister of Health, Dr Ramsammy, shared that "by criminalizing suicide, a stigma is attached to anyone who commits the act and his family who survive" (para. 1), and as a result, "additional trauma is placed on those affected" (para. 1). Dr Ramsammy also said that not all attempted suicides end up at a health care facility and when they do "the families sometimes succeed in getting the cooperation of the health worker to keep the incident quiet, because of the stigma attached to it" (para. 1).

It is probable that concerns for privacy based on Dr Ramsammy's comments may elucidate the reason Guyana's Ministry of Public Health Statistical Department had been extremely reluctant in providing me with access to key statistical research data. However, for the future, there is a need for Governmental institutions and other entities to share more information and collaborate with researchers and academics so that they can do an effective job. As a result, recruiting participants for the research initially posed a challenge. In terms of limitations, it is also recognized that collected interview data was based on the participants' perspectives, how they made meaning of their own life experiences, and the perspectives may be open to personal biases.

Summary

This chapter introduced the phenomenon of regional Indo-Guyanese suicides, based on statistics provided by PAHO/WHO, the Guyana Police Force and Guyana's Ministry of Public Health Statistics Units. I provided a brief overview of the Indo-Guyanese background, including their migration from India. In this chapter I looked at the destructive nature of suicide and presented a statement of the problem as well as my research plan to help mitigate suicides. The chapter also identified the scope and limitations of the study, including the challenges posed when accessing research participants because of the stigma and legally punitive elements attached to suicide.

As a result of the latter factors, I highlighted how suicides were underreported. I also looked at past research on suicides in Guyana and the infamous Jonestown suicides of 1978. The issue of subjectivity was highlighted as regards to the potential for participant bias. In Chapter 2, I will look at the context for my research on the Indo-Guyanese suicide phenomenon.

REFERENCE LIST

Edwards, D. (2016). Suicide in Guyana: A Sociological Analysis. Retrieved from http://guyfolkfest.org/wp-content/uploads/2016/04/Duane-Edwards-Sucide-in-Guyana-A-Sociological-Analysis.pdf

Giddens, S. (2007). Suicide: Coping in a changing world. NY: ReadHowYouWant.

Gould, M. S. (1990). Suicide clusters and media exposure.

Guyana. Bureau of Statistics. (2012). 2012 Population and Housing Census. Retrieved from https://www.statisticsguyana.gov.gy/census.html Final_2012_Census_Compendium2.pdf

Guyana Chronicle Staff Reporter. (2010, August 2). Suicide is not a crime says Health Minister. The Guyana Chronicle. Retrieved from http://guyanachronicle.com/2010/08/02/suicide-is-not-a-crime-says-health-minister

Guyana. Ministry of Legal Affairs. (2012). Laws of Guyana: Criminal Law (Offences) Act Chapter 8:01 Act 18 of 1893.Retrieved from http://mola.gov.gy/information/laws-of-guyana/903-chapter-00801-criminal-law-offences/file

Guyana. Ministry of Public Health. (2014). *National Suicide Prevention Plan: A National Suicide Prevention Strategy for Guyana (2015–2020)* [Brochure]. Guyana: Pan American Health Organization.

Guyana. Ministry of Public Health. (2015). *National Mental Health Action Plan (2015–2020)* [Brochure]. Guyana: Pan American Health Organization.

Henry, P. A. (2015). Agrochemicals, suicide ideation and social responsibility. *Issues in Social Science*, 3(2), 61.

Kilduff, M. and Javers, R. (1978). *The Suicide Cult: The inside story of the Peoples Temple sect and the massacre in Guyana.* NYC: Bantam books.

Mangar, T. (2007). East Indian Immigration, 1838–1917. *Guyana Chronicle*. Retrieved from http://www.landofsixpeoples.com/news702/nc0705062.html

Moore, R. (2008). Jonestown in Literature: Caribbean Reflections on a Tragedy. *Literature and Theology*, 23(1), 69-83.

Nock, M. K., Borges, G., Bromet, E. J., Cha, C. B., Kessler, R. C., & Lee, S. (2008). Suicide and suicidal behavior. *Epidemiologic reviews*, 30(1), 133–154.

Stephenson, D. (ed.) (2005). *Dear People: Remembering Jonestown: Selections from the Peoples Temple Collection at the California Historical Society.* Heyday Books.

Tøllefsen, I. M., Hem, E. and Ekeberg, Ø. (2012). The reliability of suicide statistics: a systematic review. *BMC psychiatry*, 12(1), 9.

World Bank. (2018). World Bank Country and Lending Groups. Retrieved from https://datahelpdesk.worldbank.org/knowledgebase/articles/906519-world-bank-country-and-lending-groups

World Health Organization. (2014). *Preventing suicide: A global imperative* [Brochure]. World Health Organization.

World Health Organization. (2018). Suicide. Retrieved from https://www.who.int/news-room/fact-sheets/detail/suicide

CHAPTER 2
INDO-GUYANESE CONTEXT

"Culture provides coping strategies to individuals; as civilization
advances many of these coping mechanisms are lost, unclothing the
genetic predisposition of vulnerable groups."
(Maharajh & Abdool, 2005)

Introduction

This chapter provides the context for research on the regional Indo-Guyanese
suicides. The chapter looks at relevant historical, demographical, and ongoing
suicidality information, as well as highlighting the study's transformational
value. My interest in the Indo-Guyanese suicide phenomenon was triggered
by what appeared to me to be an unusually large number of suicide cases that
were publicized by the media during the period 2015–2016. I was even more
concerned when I considered the high suicidality in relation to Guyana's
population size of 746,955 people.

Historical Background

Guyana is the only English-speaking country in South America and shares
cultural and historical bonds with the Anglophone Caribbean. Guyana's two
largest ethnic groups are the Afro-Guyanese (descendants of African slaves)
and the Indo-Guyanese (descendants of Indian indentured laborers), who
together comprise about three quarters of Guyana's population... Guyana's
emigration rate is among the highest in the world – more than 55% of its
citizens reside abroad (IndexMundi, 2018, para. 26).

Guyana's Bureau of Statistics (2012) states that five of Guyana's six distinct ethnic groups are

a direct result of historical immigration policy based on the country's colonial past. The population, therefore, comprises groups of persons with nationality backgrounds from Europe (Whites and Portuguese), Africa, China, and India, with the Amerindians as the indigenous population. These groups of diverse nationality backgrounds have been fused together by a common language, that is, English (p. 3).

Indo-Guyanese is one of Guyana's six people groups. Indo-Guyanese are a community of Indian immigrants who, as indentured servants, started to arrive in Guyana in May 1838, after the abolition of slavery in the British West Indies (Mangar, 2007, paras. 9–11). According to Roopnarine (2012), the indentured Indians were recruited from North and South India.

The emigrants' caste and religious compositions were somewhat representative of the caste and religious compositions in India, that is, "low- and middle-caste Indians" (p. 663) of whom 84% were Hindus and 16% were Muslims and other religions (pp. 663-664). The arrival of the people, who were referred to as 'coolies' or 'East Indians,' marked the start of a five-year indentured labour system in Guyana. The immigrants were mainly placed along the eastern coastal areas of Guyana to work on the sugar plantations. This work was later extended to include rice plantations. Hard work by the low-caste labourers gave them preferential treatment over the middle- and high-caste Indians, as well as socioeconomic mobility, and caused the original status-based caste system to be reversed (pp. 671–672). At the end of the indentured period, about 32% of the East Indians returned to India while the remainder opted to stay in Guyana.

Hintzen (1989) noted those who remained in Guyana lived in concentrated racial exclusivity in villages, communities and broader geographic areas (p. 38). I believe that this apparent grouping together aligned with the desire to maintain the comfort of the Indian culture in a different environment. Indo-Guyanese have continued to live in this grouping manner in most of the eastern coastal regions today.

According to Hookumchand and Seenarine (2000), not only did the remaining East Indians stay close to their Hindu and Islam religion and the cultural links to those religions (para. 20), including the marriage patterns from India, but money, position, education and social ranking within the ethnic group were adopted as new cultural values (para. 21).

In light of historical context, I attempted to compare the occurrence of Indian suicides to Indo-Guyanese suicides. A study by Lester (2000) reported that better epidemiological studies in India and in the countries to which Indians have emigrated

> would permit the testing of hypotheses as to the differences in suicidal behavior, including the role of the availability of different methods for suicide, the role of emigration and the immigrant experience itself, the effect of being a second-generation resident (that is, born in the new home nation), and the role of religion and ethnicity (p. 252).

However, Lester (2000) proffered that, based on evidence at the time, there seems

> little that is culturally invariant in the suicidal behavior of those from the Indian subcontinent as far as we can tell, that is, the suicidal behavior of immigrants from the Indian subcontinent does not resemble the suicidal behavior in the home nations (p. 252).

Sociocultural factors are instrumental in influencing suicidal behaviour.

A possible reason for the difference in the suicidal behaviour patterns over time is presented by Maharajh and Abdool (2005) who stated that "socio-cultural factors are instrumental in influencing suicidal behaviour. These include transgenerational cultural conflicts, psycho-social problems, media exposure, unemployment, social distress, religion and family structure" (p. 736). Maharajh and Abdool (2005) argued that "Culture is an all-embracing term and defines the relationship of an individual to his environment... Culture provides coping strategies to individuals; as civilization advances many of these coping mechanisms are lost, unclothing the genetic predisposition of vulnerable groups" (Maharajh & Abdool, 2005, p. 736).

I believe as the cultural environment changes, some people's attitudes and inter-relationships will change. I do not expect that old values, beliefs and norms within a group will perpetuate indefinitely. I believe that cultural change takes much longer to occur when a group, especially the older members from within the group, intentionally seeks to maintain the same old habits, values, beliefs and norms through clustering and exclusivity. To enable their personal, even psychological, needs to be met, new entrants to the group who force cultural change are in danger of creating sociocultural conflict. Therefore, sociocultural factors can influence suicidal behaviour. My belief aligns with Maharajh and Abdool's (2005) comments that:

> Cultural change takes much longer to occur when a group, especially the older members from within the group, intentionally seeks to maintain the same old habits, values, beliefs and norms through clustering and exclusivity.

> The effect of culture on human behaviour is equivocal with opposing views of both protective and destructive tendencies. Culture may provide a support system to an individual's vulnerability and defences related to ego-functioning, or on the other hand, may perpetuate an ecologically unhealthy environment. Often, the transgenerational loss of the old culture will result in conflicts between the mores of the traditional culture and the expectations of the modernizing society. Thus, renunciation of the old culture without assimilation of the new predisposes individuals to behavioural disturbances such as suicide. (pp. 736–737)

Scocco and Toffol (2012) state that the loss of culture may be associated with the fear of losing self-identity and it is not unusual for immigrants to concentrate in some city areas to maintain their own traditions (p. 13). If their children and grandchildren encouraged assimilation and therefore 'forced' dilution into the home culture, the change can cause suicide (p. 13). Therefore, Scocco and Toffol (2012) claim, "suicide is more common in ethnic minorities and in immigrants" (p. 13).

Suicide has historically been a part of the Indian experience, with attempted suicide, as in Guyana, being an offence under the Indian Penal Code. Somasundaram (2012) notes that India's total average yearly suicides of 123,000, "is extremely high" (p. 422). Suicides in the southern states of

Suicide has historically been a part of the Indian experience, with attempted suicide, as in Guyana, being an offence under the Indian Penal Code.

India and West Bengal are among the highest rates in the world, with Pondicherry having a suicide rate of 58.3 per 100 000 (p. 422). Many of the early emigrants from India to Guyana (called British Guiana at that time) came from Calcutta in West Bengal (Roopnarine, 2012, pp. 662–663).

Trotz (2003) describes how during the indentureship period in Guyana, there was a disparity in the sex ratio, thought to be either as a result of single women reluctant to migrate from India or resulting from the request by colonial planters for the need for only able-bodied labourers (p. 15). Another possible reason was that "respectable women did not emigrate from India" (p. 18). Male violence against women was "visible and extreme," with a number of Indian women being murdered (p. 17). According to Trotz (2003):

> Men remained wedded to their 'traditional cultural' ideas of superiority, it was disreputable and immoral women who became further emboldened under indentureship, who rebelled against their subordination to Indian men, and who ultimately paid for it with their lives. The manner of their rebellion was represented in colonial terms as a display of moral laxity; according to this logic, women could not escape responsibility for their own demise (p. 18).

As shown in this chapter, various studies have provided a number of precipitating or predisposing factors for the cause of Indian suicides; however, my study intends to determine perspective on the Indo-Guyanese suicide phenomenon by certainly acknowledging the historical background but allowing the stories shared by interview participants to provide factors based on the participants' own lived experiences. Because the regional Indo-Guyanese suicidality is a phenomenon, it is important to explore Guyana's regional geographic and demographic profile.

Geographical and Demographical Descriptions

Guyana is a mainland which shares its land borders with Suriname, Brazil and Venezuela in South America. According to Guyana's Bureau of Statistics (2012), the present population of 746,955 people is comprised of "six main heterogeneous ethnic groups apart from the 'Mixed Heritage' which derived from a combination of any of the primary groups, a consequence of intermarriage between the groups over time."

Guyana's Bureau of Statistics (2012) census reported that the largest nationality sub-group is Indo-Guyanese, comprising 39.8% of the total population (p. 3). Data from the census is shown in Table 2 and focuses on the percentage of Indo-Guyanese in the regions of interest to this study. Essentially, the Indo-Guyanese live mainly in clusters along the north-eastern coastland of Guyana where very many continue to be involved in the nation's sugar and rice production.

Table 2

Percentage of Indo-Guyanese in Region

Region	% Indo-Guyanese in Region
2	45
3	60
4	35
5	55
6	66

Although my main research focus is on the high suicidality during the period 2010 to 2016, a brief look at some recent examples shows that the Indo-Guyanese suicide phenomenon still continues.

Current Situation

WHO (2018) statistics dashboard of the latest suicide mortality rate as of 2016, showed that Guyana had the third highest suicide mortality rate in the world with 29.2 per 100 000 population, behind Russian Federation 31.0 and Lithuania 31.9 per 100 000 population (n.p.).

Additionally, WHO's (2018) statistics dashboard for the Americas shows that Guyana's suicide mortality rate is the highest for the Americas, which has a regional average suicide rate of 9.8 per 100 000 population, and it is higher than the global average suicide rate of 10.6 per 100 000 (n.p.). Guyana's suicide rate has decreased from its 2012 and 2014's highest global rates, however when considering that Guyana has a population of 746,955, less than one million people, the 2016 result is still relatively high.

Suicides are continuing to occur irrespective of age and continue to devastate family-member survivors who struggle to find answers after the sudden deaths. In a suicide, ("Boy, 15, commits Suicide," 2017), a 15-year old Indo-Guyanese boy ended his life as a result of his 12-year-old alleged girlfriend being crushed to death by a falling house in which she was staying with a family member. A young student, also 15 years old ("Mae's student, 15, dies after ingesting poison," 2019), committed suicide after first distributing suicide notes to teachers and other students.

There have been a reduced number of media-reported suicides over the last months of 2017. Fraser (2017), a legal professional, requested the creation of a Suicide Reporting Act to enable news on suicides to be reported "in a controlled and responsible manner." According to Fraser:

> Almost each day when Guyanese open the local newspapers they are bombarded with news that someone from their own community facing circumstances and hardships very similar to theirs, is dead as a result of suicide. And further, they get a good idea from the reports, in pictures if not in words, as to the methods used to commit the act. I propose that a Bill be drafted and introduced to the Parliament to curtail the reporting of deaths as suicides or suspected suicides, whether by media entities or members of the public, before the Coroner deems the death to be a suicide. The Bill will also guide reports of deaths, whether emanating from media entities or members of the public, so that they do not reflect even the suspicion that a death may have been

a suicide, before the Coroner deems the death to be a possible suicide (paras. 2,3).

Fraser's call for legal intervention triggers an awareness of the local, national, and cultural factors that impact Indo-Guyanese suicide epidemiology. I believe that Fraser is prompting the Guyana Government to not simply intervene legally to curb media reporting, but to look at how suicide is perceived, the style and possibly the intentional impact-reporting of suicides and attempted suicides by the media. Although impact-reporting brings attention to the problem, it may guide individuals' worldviews and even contribute to the extension of the suicide problem. I believe that Fraser is also asking the Guyana Government to look at the way key institutions' personnel, particularly first responders and clinicians, record and deal with deaths. If the issues surrounding suicide are not dealt with effectively by all parties concerned, there remains the potential for persistent underreporting as a result of the stigma attached to suicide; false diagnoses; suicide contagion, and the general acceptance of suicide as an everyday occurrence in the small nation of Guyana.

Guyana's Public Health Ministry has joined with PAHO to produce the five-year National Suicide Prevention Plan 2015–2020 for use mainly by mental health clinicians. A personal conversation with the Director of Mental Health Unit, Dr Util Richmond-Thomas, (U. Richmond-Thomas, personal communication, March 2017) revealed that in an effort to mitigate suicide, there will be a transitioning of the mental health care system from institutionalization to community-based. Dr Thomas also stated that the National Suicide Prevention Plan 2015–2020 and the National Mental Health Action Plan 2015–2020 are guiding the work of the Mental Health Unit ensuring health care workers are trained to deal with conditions such as depression and suicide. Many will be interested in the level of success of Guyana's National Suicide Prevention Plan 2015–2020.

A small number of NGOs in Guyana are currently working within some communities to provide prevention and postvention therapy such as counselling, but the stigma attached to suicide and the

> The stigma attached to suicide and the community's protective nature towards persons who have attempted suicide as well as to family-member survivors, sometimes hamper efficient and effective support.

community's protective nature towards persons who have attempted suicide as well as to family-member survivors, sometimes hamper efficient and effective support (U. Richmond-Thomas, personal communication, March 2017).

Suicide is a global issue and Bertolote and Fleischmann (2002) noted that based on the world trend, suicide will reach an annual figure of 1.53 million in 2020 (p. 6). I believe that in order to get a significant decrease in the number of suicides, it is essential to study the root cause of the problem before appropriate interventions can be implemented, and these interventions should be made based on their applicability to the population being studied. My study focused on how to reduce Indo-Guyanese suicides, thereby bringing transformation to the lives of one of Guyana's largest people groups.

Attaining Transformation

Rogers (2010) said, "It is one thing for an individual to decide to adopt a new idea, quite a different thing to put the innovation to use, as problems in exactly how to use the innovation crop up at the implementation stage" (p. 179). This study highlights the Indo-Guyanese suicide phenomenon. Most, if not all, Guyanese are aware of the suicide phenomenon. Finding an appropriate way to effectively mitigate the problem is essential in order to bring transformation to the affected families, communities and to the nation.

> It is one thing for an individual to decide to adopt a new idea, quite a different thing to put the innovation to use, as problems in exactly how to use the innovation crop up at the implementation stage.

The interviews with suicide attempters and family-member survivors provided a platform for participants to share and make meaning of their lived experiences. I believe that sharing their experiences in a safe, confidential, and non-judgmental environment offered some transformation to participants. Many of the participants came from a place of not being understood and were trying to address the unanswered questions as to the reason a loved one opted to die by suicide.

Grounded theory was used to process the interview data and give meaning to the Indo-Guyanese suicide phenomenon. The theorization process was inductive, shedding light on the suicide phenomenon and bringing transformation through enlightenment of the potential adopters in the consultation process. Potential adopters were informed of the research findings in a consultation meeting.

An aim of the consultation meeting was to diffuse the findings to diverse agencies, enabling them to start the collaboration process and to determine the next steps forward in mitigating Indo-Guyanese suicides. To ensure that practical transformation was produced, the research findings were primarily disbursed and discussed at a consultation meeting with policymakers at local, regional, and national levels.

Another aim of the consultation meeting was to determine necessary suicide interventions and postventions using proactive ways and multi-sectorial, holistic approaches. The approaches involved helping to raise awareness through diverse agencies; providing relevant training to key personnel; developing and implementing new strategies; updating existing strategies, policies, and legal framework; and, policymakers implementing new safeguarding organizational structures to protect at-risk persons. Most importantly having continuous conversations and collaboration to ensure there is an ongoing rigorous approach towards mitigating Indo-Guyanese suicides.

After the consultation, my organization Ephrathah, which has a mission to educate, guide, and empower individuals, provided counselling for 40 at-risk persons in one of the five regions. Ephrathah will continue to provide effective and relevant support where needed in terms of suicide education, training, and counselling. Overall, my research provides a platform for the discussion of how to construct effective and transformative interventions to mitigate the suicide phenomenon.

Summary

In this chapter, I have provided historical, geographic, and demographic information to elucidate the Indo-Guyanese context. I have looked at indentureship and highlighted the propensity for regional racial exclusivity in the lives of the East Indians, now Indo-Guyanese, as they settled in Guyana. The chapter also explored sociocultural and transgenerational conflicts and their relationship to suicidal behavior. I have looked at how media reporting can create suicide contagion and how this contagion can be prevented by legal intervention and responsible media reporting. In looking at the current situation, I provided recent examples of Indo-Guyanese suicides. I concluded with the practicability and importance of the study in its attempt to bring transformation by enlightening potential adopters in a consultative process.

In Chapter 3, I will describe events surrounding a suicide which took place. A pseudo-name is given to the victim. I was given permission to tell the story by family-member survivors, with the hope that it will encourage persons experiencing suicide ideation to seek professional help.

REFERENCE LIST

Bertolote, J. M., & Fleischmann, A. (2002). A global perspective in the epidemiology of suicide. *Suicidologi*, 7(2), 6-8.

Boy, 15, commits Suicide Days after House crushes Girlfriend. (2017, August 23). Kaieteur News. Retrieved from https://www.kaieteurnewsonline.com/2017/08/23/boy-15-commits-suicide-days-after-house-crushes-girlfriend/

Guyana. Bureau of Statistics. (2012). 2012 Population and Housing Census. Retrieved from https://www.statisticsguyana.gov.gy/census.html Final_2012_Census_Compendium2.pdf

Hintzen, P. C. (1989). *The Costs of Regime Survival: Racial Mobilization, Elite Domination and Control of the State in Guyana and Trinidad.* England: Cambridge University Press.

Hookumchand, G. and Seenarine, M. (2000). Conflict between East-Indian and Blacks in Trinidad and Guyana socially, economically and politically. *Guyana News and Information.* Retrieved from http://www.guyana.org/features/conflicts_indiansandblacks.html

IndexMundi. (2018). Guyana Demographics Profile 2018. Retrieved from https://www.indexmundi.com/guyana/demographics_profile.html

Lester, D. (2000). Suicide in emigrants from the Indian subcontinent. *Transcultural psychiatry*, 37(2), 243-254.

Mae's student, 15, dies after ingesting poison. (2019, January 25). *Stabroek News.* Retrieved from https://www.stabroeknews.com/2019/news/guyana/01/25/maes-student-15-dies-after-ingesting-poison/

Maharajh, H. D. and Abdool, P. S. (2005). Cultural aspects of suicide. *The Scientific World Journal*, 5, 736-746.

Mangar, T. (2007). East Indian Immigration, 1838–1917. *Guyana Chronicle.*

Retrieved from http://www.landofsixpeoples.com/news702/nc0705062.html

Rogers, E. M. (2010). *Diffusion of innovations*. NYC: Simon and Schuster.

Roopnarine, L. (2012). Regulations and Remittances from British Indian Indentured Guianese. *Comparative Studies of South Asia, Africa and the Middle East*, 32(3), 662–673.

Scocco, P. and Toffol, E. (2012). Loss, Hopelessness and Suicide. In *Suicide from a global perspective: psychosocial approaches*. New York: Nova Science, pp. 11–17.

Somasundaram, D. (2012). Suicide and Society in India. *Asian Studies Review*, 36(3), 422–423.

Trotz, D. A. (2003). Behind the banner of culture? Gender, "race," and the family in Guyana. *New West Indian Guide/Nieuwe West-Indische Gids*, 77(1-2), 5–29.

World Health Organization. (2018). World Health Statistics data visualizations dashboard. Retrieved from http://apps.who.int/gho/data/node.sdg.3-4-viz-2?lang=en

PART 2
PSYCHOLOGY OF SUICIDES

CHAPTER 3
A COMPLETED SUICIDE

"The loss of a loved one to death is widely recognized as a challenging
stressor event, one that increases risk for the development of many
psychiatric conditions. One key risk factor is the mode of death."
(Jordan, 2008)

Introduction

This chapter details an actual Indo-Guyanese suicide as described by family-member survivors. I also highlight some key aspects of the suicide as a point of reference for discussions in later chapters. Due to the sensitive nature of the contents of this chapter, I have not used any real names and I have adjusted physical descriptions and locations so that no one can be identified. I have been granted permission to publish this story so that readers can learn from it, recognize some risk factors and help to mitigate suicide.

A Completed Suicide Described by Family-Member Survivors

Ram was a sole trader, doing multiple jobs so as to eke out a living to maintain his family. He was 42 years old on the day he hung himself on a tree. He died alone in the early morning hours after he had spent part of his last night pacing the garden pathway and having suicidal ideation.

Ram's Last Night
According to a survivor, earlier that night Ram was jovial, doing and saying 'weird' things. He did not engage in the things he would normally do such as sitting and watching television outside of the house. Instead, he went inside the house and sat on a sofa next to his sister and engaged in jovial reflections

of his life. During the conversation, Ram repeatedly asked when a close relative, who was working a very long distance away at the time, would be returning home. The relative was expected home on the same day of Ram's suicide. Instead of a written suicide note, Ram left a voice message for one of his close friends. Apart from leaving the one song he repeatedly played on the night he committed suicide, Ram deliberately cleared the contents of his telephone. No one could fully decipher Ram's final thoughts on that fateful night.

Previous Attempt and Consequence

The fatal suicide was Ram's second attempt at suicide. Ram first attempted suicide two years earlier as a result of experiencing intimate partner violence (IPV). The physical abuse from the IPV was violent enough to leave obvious marks on his body. The first suicide attempt failed because a family-member rescued Ram as he attempted to hang himself. As a result of the attempted suicide, and in accordance to the law in Guyana, Ram was immediately imprisoned. To find where Ram was imprisoned, his sister had to search many police stations before she was able to locate him. On his early release, Ram stayed with his sister for two years but finally decided to return to his home. His return home was two months before his death.

His sister reflected that Ram was feeling very stressed over the challenging domestic situation, which included having to stop an arranged marriage for one of his young children. As a result of the stressful family events, Ram became very depressed and started to smoke heavily.

Life-changing Event

A few days prior to his suicide Ram had received a court summons with the probability of a restraining order imposed on him to prevent him from accessing his family home, where his wife and two children lived. Two days after receiving the summons he returned to stay with his sister, telling her "I am only here for 3 to 4 days." His sister did not understand the full extent of what Ram was saying, especially when he also told her he was going to Surinam, then later shared that he was going into the 'interior' (the areas outside of Guyana's coastal plain) to work.

After receiving the summons, Ram was adamant that he was not going to court to face the likelihood of a restraining order. He did not want to be evicted from his home. He wanted to be with his children.

Planning the suicide

Some days before his suicide, Ram had told several non-family persons, mostly his customers, of his plan to end his life, but no one took him seriously or reported it. Ram's sister reflected that because they were so closely related, he felt she would try to stop him from committing suicide. Four days before he died he was seen giving away his clothes and other personal possession.

Ram had made his decision to commit suicide. On his last night, he wanted his sister and nieces to experience his jovial side when he sat with them.

After the suicide

Ram left family-member survivors who felt deep hurt and loss, questioning why he would choose to commit suicide, and by such a method as hanging. They asked themselves why Ram did not choose to talk to someone instead of choosing to commit suicide. The neighbours were in shock when they heard of the incident and wanted to know why Ram had committed suicide. When asked what was causing the hurt, all the family members being interviewed unanimously blamed themselves for not being able to prevent the suicide and for not recognizing the signs leading up to Ram's death. Ram had given money to two young persons in the community and told them they would not receive any more gifts from him. Days before his suicide, he had also cleared all his debts. No one had taken any notice of his actions. A week after Ram's suicide, he was cremated.

First Responders

After Ram was found hanging by family members, the police were informed and they arrived about half an hour later. A male police officer asked for the family to get someone to cut Ram down from the tree. A petite female relative volunteered to take him down but another male relative stepped in and brought Ram down. The police later used a family member's mobile phone to call the morgue because none of them had credits on their mobiles phones to make the call. Ram's family was never offered bereavement counselling.

Key Factors in the Completed Suicide

A number of issues are presented in this suicide, which is not unusual and highlights the complexities that the person investigating such a case will have to manage. I have presented the issues below in no order of priority and some of these issues will be looked at in more detail in Chapter 4.

Basic Profile of the Indo-Guyanese suicider
At age 42, Ram fell into the category of persons who were committing suicide most frequently in Guyana. According to Guyana's Ministry of Public Health (2015), suicide is the fourth leading cause of death among persons aged 25 to 44 (p. 20). Figure 9 also shows the high consistency of more Indo-Guyanese males committing suicide over females for the period 2010–2016.

Method of Suicide
Hanging is the method of choice of many male suicide victims. Denning, Yeates, Key and Cox (2000) found that "Women who commit suicide use less violent methods, such as drugs and carbon monoxide poisoning, than do men, who more often use violent methods such as guns and hanging" (p. 282).

Previous Suicide Attempts
A previous suicide attempt is a risk factor for suicide. According to Teasdale (1988), "Beck theorized that previous suicidal experience sensitizes suicide-related thoughts and behaviours such that they later become more accessible and active." Where there has been a history of previous suicide attempts, it is most likely that the attempter will try until the act is completed.

Life-changing Incident – Family Conflict / Domestic Abuse
Discordant or conflictual family relationships can affect mental health. Ram was a victim of IPV and other domestic situations which caused him to experience stress and depression. The true amount of IPV is unknown and particularly where the abused is male.

According to Barnett, Miller-Perrin and Perrin (2010), "research about cohabitors …is meager" (p. 256) and "It is worth noting that when couples complete surveys or interviews, their reports of IPV do not customarily agree" (p. 260). They also state that "IPV probably does occur more frequently

CHAPTER 4
INSIGHTS INTO THE SUICIDAL MIND

Suicide is man's great retreat from life. He has recourse to it when he
feels no longer able to endure suffering in the present or pain in the
future. It is therefore a failure of adaptation and constitutes a final regression from reality. The motives underlying suicidal acts are numerous and
complex. It is impossible to ascertain them with any degree of certainty
unless we are intimately acquainted with the patient's psychic life.
(Crichton-Miller, 1931)

Introduction

This chapter reviews major sources on suicide in my quest to provide understanding of the reasons people commit or attempt suicide, and the resultant
grief of family-member survivors. I compare various sources, at times com-
menting on whether I agree or disagree with some of the views.

I, firstly, provide a general review of the epidemiology of suicides and suicide attempts, including underreporting, and a brief exploration of the mental
and emotional conditions associated with suicide. Secondly, I look at the
Indo-Guyanese suicide phenomenon by focusing on familial, social and religious factors to provide a better understanding of the people group. Thirdly,
I look at literature that relates to features of the qualitative research in terms
of the platform provided to hear the
stories of participants, the sample of
suicide attempters, and family-member survivors. Finally, I look at studies
on grounded theory, recognizing the
potential for researcher bias as well as
participants' bias.

Suicide is an outcome of
many factors which relate
to the individual's lived
experiences and very
often include sociocultural
interactions.

Suicide is an outcome of many

37

factors which relate to the individual's lived experiences and very often include sociocultural interactions. When someone commits suicide family, friends and even the community may be devastated. When someone has tried and failed to commit suicide, without the proper help they may spend the rest of their lives dealing with the damage caused by the failed attempt. For many the physical and emotional scars from the trauma may be too much to cope with and they often end up repeating the suicide attempt, until they succeed in killing themselves.

I have wondered at the reason people commit suicide. I have also wondered what can be the workings of human minds that would lead them to attempt suicide, in full knowledge of suicide's potential lethality and the resultant impact on families and communities. There are many proffered theories concerning suicide and loss from suicide. However, there is not much published research available on the Indo-Guyanese suicide experience, which has seen Guyana having the highest global suicide rates for 2012 and 2014 and also significantly, most of the suicides were committed by Indo-Guyanese (Ministry of Public Health, 2014, pp. 8, 13). WHO (2018) suicide dashboard shows that Guyana has the third highest global suicide rate of 29.2 per 100,000 (n.p.).

Epidemiology of Suicides and Suicide Attempts

WHO's (2014) first Global Report on suicide stated that every year approximately one person commits suicide every 40 seconds. Global epidemiology of suicide and attempted suicide indicates that an estimated 804,000 suicide deaths occurred worldwide in 2012, representing an annual global age-standardized suicide rate of 11.4 per 100 000 population; and for every suicide there are many more people who attempt suicide every year. The report also

> Global epidemiology of suicide and attempted suicide indicates that an estimated 804,000 suicide deaths occurred worldwide in 2012, representing an annual global age-standardized suicide rate of 11.4 per 100 000 population; and for every suicide there are many more people who attempt suicide every year.

stated that a prior suicide attempt is the single most important risk factor for suicide in the general population.

Hutchinson, Daisley, Simmons and Gordon (1991) conducted

> An epidemiological evaluation... on 270 patients who died at the General Hospital, Port-of-Spain after presenting with deliberate self-poisoning between January, 1986 and June, 1990. The cause of death was confirmed by autopsy and toxicological analysis... It was found that the male to female ratio was 2.7:1. East Indians accounted for 54.4%, Africans 42.0%, people of mixed ethnic origin 3% and Caucasians 0.6% [of suicides]... "Lovers' quarrels" (35.4% of cases), psychiatric illness (27.8% of cases) and family disputes (27% of cases) were reported as the most frequent precipitating events in suicide. East Indians predominated in those suicides precipitated by "lovers' quarrels" and family disputes, accounting for 63.2% and 58.9% of these cases, respectively... Paraquat was the most popular poison used in 63.7% of the suicidal cases, and other agrochemicals were used in 20% of cases.

Hutchinson and colleagues' research shows the multi-faceted nature of suicide and also provide some key statistics on the East Indians in Trinidad suicidality.

Bertolote and Fleischmann (2002) examined suicide data provided by WHO's Member States, looking at gender, age and the prevailing religion to present global suicide rates from 1950 to 1998 and trends to 2020. Based on the data, it was estimated that from current trends, in 2020, 1.53 million people will die from suicide, and 10–20 times more people will attempt suicide worldwide, an average of one suicide death every 20 seconds. The highest numbers of suicides were found in Asia, with almost 30% of all suicides being committed in China and India alone (pp. 6–7).

Moscicki (2001) provided a review of epidemiologic studies of completed and attempted suicides and also discussed interventions. Unlike Bertolote and Fleischmann, Moscicki focused his research mainly on data from the United States (US) in 1998 and looked at risk factors for both suicides and attempted

> In 2020, 1.53 million people will die from suicide, and 10–20 times more people will attempt suicide worldwide, an average of one suicide death every 20 seconds.

> Hopelessness is "the perception that one's negative life's circumstances are unlikely to improve, or that there is no way to solve an important problem or escape psychological pain".

suicides. He found that the outcome of suicide was based on a number of risk factors, which included mental disorders, familial risk factors such as a dysfunctional family and negative parenting, stressful life events such as the loss of a loved one or rejection, contagion and hopelessness (pp. 315–318). Cornette, Mathias, Marsh, DeRoon-Cassini and Dougherty (2012) define *hopelessness* as "the perception that one's negative life's circumstances are unlikely to improve, or that there is no way to solve an important problem or escape psychological pain" (p. 3). Contagion occurs where exposure to suicidal behaviours influences vulnerable persons to want to commit suicide. As discussed earlier, there is pressure on the Guyanese media to ensure responsible reporting in order to avoid contagion driven Indo-Guyanese suicides (Fraser, 2017).

Nock et al. (2008) note that suicidal behaviour is a leading cause of injury and death worldwide, and information about the epidemiology of such behavior is important for policy-making and prevention (p. 133). According to them, most epidemiologic research on suicidal behavior has focused on patterns and correlates of prevalence (p. 133) such as biological factors and trends. Bertolote and Fleischmann's global suicide research followed the same focus of patterns and correlates (p. 6). I perceive the results of these studies to be helpful; however, Nock and colleagues suggest that in order to decrease the large number of suicides, "new studies must incorporate recent advances in survey methods and clinical assessment" (p. 133). The importance of clinical assessment cannot be minimized, particularly if strategic interventions to mitigate suicide, and the resultant suffering caused by suicide, accompany the process. My research focused on two strategic assessment options. Firstly, I used grounded theory to analyze interview data and produce the research findings. Secondly, clinicians assessed the findings at a consultation forum in order to develop appropriate interventions.

> Suicidal behaviour is a leading cause of injury and death worldwide, and information about the epidemiology of such behavior is important for policy-making and prevention.

The high number of suicides highlighted for India prompted me to consider if there were any possible links between the high rate of Indo-Guyanese suicides and the Indian high suicide rates. Radhakrishnan and Andrade (2012) state that "An understanding of suicide in the Indian context calls for an appreciation of the literary, religious, and cultural ethos of the subcontinent because tradition has rarely permeated the lives of people for as long as it has in India" (p. 2). According to their study, in ancient India, suicides were celebrated if they were committed to avoid shame and disgrace.

> The Vedas permit suicide for religious reasons and consider that the best sacrifice was that of one's own life.... Sati, where a woman immolated herself on the pyre of her husband rather than live the life of a widow and Jauhar, in which Rajput women killed themselves to avoid capture and humiliation at the hands of the invading Muslim armies, were both a part of Hindu tradition (p. 2).

However, according to Radhakrishnan and Andrade (p. 2) the Hindus' "Bhagavad Gita condemns suicide for selfish reasons and posits such a death by suicide cannot have 'shraddha,' the all-important last rites," while the Hindus' Upanishads also condemn suicide and state that "he who takes his own life will enter the sunless areas covered by impenetrable darkness after death" (p. 3).

In India, Hindus believe that suicides and attempted suicides must be done in the home because, according to Sharma and Gopalakrishna (1978):

> a person will not reach heaven after his death unless certain religious rites have been performed and the body has been religiously disposed of...a suicidal act may be viewed as a kind of an assault on the community and arouse feelings of guilt in significant persons in the family and society (p. 16).

In Guyana, some Indo-Guyanese suicides, including three from my research, have occurred in the victims' homes, but many have occurred outside of the home, including Guyana's famous Kaieteur Falls. In the case of the latter, victims have had to board a plane and travel for an hour to reach the Falls, possibly fully cognizant that they were making their final earthly journey ("Second suicide in two months at Guyana's Kaieteur Falls," 2015).

41

Cognition and Suicide

To understand what drives an individual to commit suicide, it is helpful to understand the cognition that precedes suicide ideation and behaviours. According to Cornette et al. (2012), "aspects of social and neurocognition are among the most salient risk factors for suicide, and include our perceptions of ourselves and others, and how adept we are at solving interpersonal dilemmas" (p. 3). They have proposed certain cognitive factors which influence the decision to commit suicide (pp. 3–6).These factors include feelings of hopelessness; ruminative thinking which Nolen-Hoeksema (1991) describes as repetitive, perseverative thinking about life's events, particularly focusing on the associated negative emotional states (p. 569); perfectionism which Cornette and colleagues define as the "state in which the individual determinedly pursues self-imposed, personally demanding standards, despite adverse consequences" (p. 4); poor problem-solving skills; perceived burdensomeness and thwarted belongingness; and dissociation described by Cornette and colleagues as "a disruption in the integrated functions of consciousness, memory or perception" (p. 5).

Bereaved family and friends may experience "feelings of shame, guilt, sadness and the effects of trauma, stigma and social isolation, and they seek to understand why the death occurred" (Wertheimer, 2013, p. xi). According to Scocco and Toffol (2012), "bereavement is considered to be one of the most stressful life events" (p.12) and when associated with suicide, it can lead to complicated grief, especially where there is an attempt to make meaning of the loss (p. 12). They also claim that a disruption in, or fear of losing, one's sense of self-identity caused, for example, as a result of bereavement or role transition can lead to suicide (p. 14). "Hopelessness is closely related to bereavement, role transition, culture loss and self-identity disruption since it is the common emotional reaction to all these" (p. 14).

According to McKenzie, Serfaty and Crawford (2003), environmental, individual factors, and "socio-economic stress, thwarted aspirations, racism, acculturation, culture clash with parents, loss of religious affiliations, difficulty with identity formation and loss of family and community support" (p. 101) determine the suicide risk in immigrants. In comparing the state of mind of individuals who made impulsive suicide attempts with those who made a premeditated attempt, Spokas, Wenzel, Brown, and Beck (2012) found that individuals who made an impulsive attempt were less depressed and hopeless and expected their attempts to be less lethal. However, the lethality in the impulsive attempt group was similar to the premeditated attempt (p. 1).

Hopelessness is a common thread in most of the studies in this section. I agree that hopelessness is an emotional state that can make people extremely vulnerable and also potentially susceptible to irrational behaviour, such as suicide. The interview process in my research was guided by a questionnaire instrument which included cognition checks before, during and after the suicide or suicide attempt. These checks formed part of the overall assessment strategy for the research. I believe that understanding the cognitive state of participants can determine whether the suicide attempter is likely to repeat the suicide attempt.

Van Orden et al. (2010) proposed an interpersonal theory that to "a larger extent the same mental processes underlie all forms of suicidal behavior" (p. 25), and cite three constructs as being central to suicidal behavior. Firstly, thwarted belongingness is the lack of social connectedness (p. 9) and where individuals exhibit suicidal behavior because they feel unsupported by others, and they do not support others (p. 43). Secondly, perceived burdensomeness is when individuals perceive they are a burden to persons they are in close relationship with, believing that they are flawed and a liability to others (p. 12). They may also have "affectively-laden cognitions of self-hatred" which is linked to low self-esteem, self-blame, shame, and the presentation of agitation (pp. 12–13, 44). The third construct is an acquired capability for suicide, "a multi-dimensional emergent latent variable that involves the dimensions of lowered fear of death and increased physical pain tolerance" (pp. 15–16, 45), that is, through repeating the suicidal behavior, the individual engages in increasingly more painful and fearful aspects of self-harm. This third construct clarifies the reason persons who have committed multiple suicide attempts are more likely to eventually kill themselves (p. 15), and enables exploration of the psychological pain in the lived experience of the suicide attempter.

Psychology of Suicide

There is a great deal of pain in the world today, including the unbearable psychological pain associated with suicide. Crichton-Miller (1931) notes that:

Suicide is man's great retreat from life. He has recourse to it when he feels no longer able to endure suffering in the present or pain in the future. It is therefore a failure of adaptation and constitutes a final regression from reality. (p. 239)

Suicide is man's great retreat from life.

Crichton-Miller states that it is impossible to determine the motives underlying suicidal acts unless there is understanding of the person's psychic life. The motives are placed into three categories (p. 239). The first category is physical pain, including frustration of instinctive demands. "We are probably justified in concluding, at any rate for civilized man, that he is more capable of adjusting to physical pain than to anticipatory dread of it." The second category is social sufferings and fears, where social humiliation or the fear of misdeeds being discovered is too hard to cope with. The third category is doubts and dreads pertaining to the hereafter. He states that fear of a pending situation rather than being in the actual situation drives a person to suicide (p. 240).

Like Crichton-Miller, Shneidman (1993) considered the psyche and theorized that suicide is caused by psychache, an unbearable psychological pain in the psyche or mind. He describes psychache as the "hurt, anguish, soreness, aching psychological *pain* in the psyche, the mind" (p. 145). The pain may be caused by "excessively felt shame, or guilt, or humiliation, or loneliness, or fear, or angst, or dread of growing old or of dying badly, or whatever", factors which block, thwart or frustrate certain psychological needs which are vital for the continuation of the person's life. Suicide results when the person's threshold can no longer tolerate the pain. According to him, a study of emotional feelings is critical to understanding suicidal behaviour because it is not non-psychological factors such as socioeconomic levels, nor psychiatric categories such as depression that cause suicide, but psychache caused by unmet psychological needs. Being adjustive, suicide "serves to reduce the tension of the pain related to the blocked needs."

According to Barbour (1994), many suicidal persons place themselves in situations where they are likely to die. However, they warn others of their plan or arrange to be discovered before they are dead or feel relieved when they are rescued from death. Many suicide attempters deny that their primary intention is to die but insist they do not want to live without a particular entity (p. 81).

It is helpful to consider the psychology behind various theories on suicide and the explanations surrounding suicide risk factors, however, my research aimed to investigate a specific people group and provide understanding of their lived experiences. By adhering to the tenets of grounded theory, I did not go into the research seeking to test the effects of any predefined suicide risk factors, but I allowed the analyzed interview data to provide an understanding of what motivated Indo-Guyanese to attempt or commit suicide.

Stigma and Grief of Suicide

The experience of having a loved one commit suicide is not only grievous but often stigmatized, as studies show. The stigma, as shown earlier, often has legal and religious connotation. Jordan and McIntosh (2011) claim that suicide bereavement shares the same elements of grief as any other loss, but some elements are likely to be more prominent after suicide, such as stigmatization, anger, guilt, and making sense of the suicide (pp. 303–306).

> Suicide survivors are defined as "people who are grieving after the loss of someone important to them to suicide" including the immediate family, friends, neighbours, co-workers, and entire communities.

Jordan (2015) defines suicide survivors as "people who are grieving after the loss of someone important to them to suicide" including the immediate family, friends, neighbours, co-workers, and entire communities. According to him, suicide survivors are left to wonder, "Why did they do this? Whose fault is it? Could we have done something to see it coming or prevent it? How could they do this to me/us?" (p. 349).

> Suicide survivors are left to wonder, "Why did they do this?"

He noted that there is "a growing appreciation of the psychological damage that suicide may cause to those left behind" (p. 350). There is also "substantial evidence that survivors may experience high levels of psychiatric morbidity, social alienation, and stigmatization, and longer term mental health consequences." De Groot and Kollen (2013) highlighted "Symptoms of complicated grief might contribute to the increased risk of suicide in relatives bereaved by suicide" (p. 1).

> Symptoms of complicated grief might contribute to the increased risk of suicide in relatives bereaved by suicide.

Jordan and McIntosh (2011) claimed "More stigmatization appears to be attached to people who have lost a loved one to suicide. Concern about being judged or perceived negatively by others may result in the suicide bereaved hiding the real cause of the death" (p. 303). Further, they stated that "suicide may entail a powerful rupturing of the mourner's assumptive world,

Concern about being judged or perceived negatively by others may result in the suicide bereaved hiding the real cause of the death.

including the belief that we can fully know other people" (p. 350).

This thought coincides with Crichton-Miller's, when he claimed that motives for suicides can only be discovered by getting into a person's psychic life (p. 239), attempting to decipher and provide understanding of what was in the mind of someone who attempted suicide, which was the goal of this research, done by listening to and making meaning of the participants' stories. Linked to the associated grief from suicide, Jordan (2015) stated that as a family attempts to manage the intense pain associated with their grief, they may experience tension as a result of "'coping asynchrony,' a mismatch of individual family members' coping styles that may create relational strain" (p. 354).

Motives for suicides can only be discovered by getting into a person's psychic life.

Suicides may often occur in clusters, known also as suicide contagion, a situation where one suicide triggers a number of other suicides. The contagion effect of grief, where survivors are overwhelmed by the loss of a loved one or peer, "may also have the effect of 'giving permission' to others who are unhappy" (Doka, 2014, p. 48). This effect is an important discovery particularly when considering Bertolote and Fleischmann's prediction on the rise in the global suicide trend (p. 6).

'Coping asynchrony,' a mismatch of individual family members' coping styles that may create relational strain.

To avoid suicide contagion, the media are often asked to deliver responsible reporting. WHO (2000) produced a summary of guidelines (Table 3) to enable responsible media reporting (p. 8).

Table 3

WHO (2000) guidelines for media reporting

What to do	What not to do
Work closely with health authorities in presenting the facts.	Don't publish photographs or suicide notes.
Refer to suicide as a completed suicide, not a successful one.	Don't report specific details of the method used.
Present only relevant data, on the inside pages.	Don't give simplistic reasons.
Highlight alternatives to suicide.	Don't glorify or sensationalize suicide.
Provide information on helplines and community resources.	Don't use religious or cultural stereotypes.
Publicize risk indicators and warning signs.	Don't apportion blame.

I believe if these guidelines are adhered to by the Guyanese media, particularly where suicide is sensationalized and graphic details are printed of the suicide, contagion may be prevented. Also, according to WHO (2000), the media must "Work closely with health authorities in presenting the facts" (p. 8).

According to Overholser et al. (1995), self-esteem can play an important role in suicidality, particularly in young people, "adolescents with low self-esteem who were more likely to have previously attempted suicide and were more likely to be experiencing suicidal ideation" (p. 924). *Suicidal ideation* is having thoughts about committing suicide. Overholser and colleagues describe *self-esteem* as "the global appraisal a person makes of his or her own value as a competent and worthwhile person" (p. 919).

Stigma as mentioned earlier is linked to suicide. A study by Crocker and Major (1989) shared that "although several psychological theories predict that members of stigmatized groups should have low global self-esteem, empirical research typically does not support this prediction" (p. 608). Additionally, they state that "stigmatized individuals are not merely passive victims but are frequently able actively

Self-esteem is "the global appraisal a person makes of his or her own value as a competent and worthwhile person".

47

to protect and buffer their self-esteem from prejudice and discrimination" (p. 624). I believe that any protective buffer generated by stigma may result in a further loss of voice and alienation for suicide survivors and attempters unless they possess enough resilience to cope with the consequences of stigmatization and potential social silence. An understanding of how people respond to stigma was valuable for this phenomenological research because of the stigma attached to Indo-Guyanese suicides.

Limitation of Underreporting of Suicides

Literary works have pointed towards underreporting of suicides for a number of reasons (Katz, Bolton and Sareen, 2016, p. 2). Underreporting not only implies that the number of suicides and suicide attempts reported globally are much higher (Tøllefsen et al., 2012, p. 1), but given that all of the WHO Member States do not contribute to providing suicide information, it increases the level of underreporting (Bertolote and Fleischmann, 2002, p. 6).

According to Sartorius (2012), despite the high numbers of suicides, in many countries, suicide is not treated as a major health problem and as such effective recordings of deaths by suicide are not provided (p. xv). As mentioned earlier, Tøllefsen and colleagues showed in their study that there is general underreporting of suicides and nationwide studies, and comparisons between countries are lacking. The main finding was that there is a lack of systematic assessment of the reliability of suicide statistics (p. 1). Katz et al. (2016) found reporting is affected by the

> tendency of suicides to be misclassified as undetermined intent. The decedent may have tried to mask their intentions due to stigma or to protect their family emotionally or financially. Further, there are differences in approach and methods between medical examiners and coroners and between various regions and countries. (p. 2)

Maharajh and Abdool (2005) state that low rates of suicide are reported in Muslim countries such as Pakistan, possibly due to "strict legal and religious sanctions against suicidal behavior." They conclude that "Culture, therefore, may sometimes affect the reporting rather than the suicidal act" (p. 739).

I have studied the mainly Hindu Indo-Guyanese community because of the high recorded suicide rates. However, the level of underreporting raises questions not only about the accuracy of the Indo-Guyanese suicide statistics but the statistics for the other ethnic groups. Underreporting ultimately affects the accuracy of Guyana's published national suicide rates.

Exploring the Phenomenon of Suicide among Indo-Guyanese

My research sought to provide understanding on the regional suicide phenomenon occurring within the Indo-Guyanese population. To develop and evaluate theory, concepts concerning that theory must be identified, analyzed, and defined. The concepts may include psychological, familial, sociocultural, and religious factors.

Guyana Ministry of Public Health (2014) published its National Suicide Prevention Plan for 2015 to 2020, which reports the increasingly high rate of suicide in Guyana. The plan highlights that every year in Guyana, one person commits suicide every day and a half (p. 5). Figure 4 shows total suicides versus total Indo-Guyanese suicides in Guyana for the period 2010 to 2016.

TOTAL SUICIDES IN GUYANA vs INDO-GUYANESE SUICIDES 2010–2016

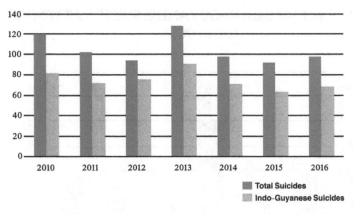

FIGURE 4. Total suicides in Guyana vs Indo-Guyanese suicides 2010-2016

There is an estimated ratio of 20 to 25 cases of attempted suicides for every suicide death (p. 18). Figure 5 shows total suicides versus total suicide attempts in Guyana for the period 2010 to 2016.

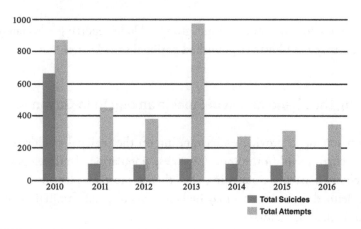

FIGURE 5. Total suicides vs total attempts 2010-2016

Indo-Guyanese account for more than 80% of reported suicides in Guyana, and most of these suicides are in the North East Coastal Regions 2 to 6 (p. 17). Indo-Guyanese accounted for more than 50% of reported attempted suicides and most of the attempted suicides were also in the same coastal Regions 2 to 6 (p. 18). Figure 6 shows female versus male Indo-Guyanese suicide attempts for the period 2010 through 2016.

FEMALE vs MALE INDO-GUYANESE SUICIDE ATTEMPTS 2010-2016

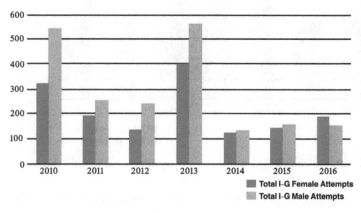

FIGURE 6. Female vs male Indo-Guyanese suicide attempts 2010-2016

Guyana reported in its National Mental Health Plan for 2015 to 2020 that the WHO (2014) Global Suicide Report recorded Guyana as the country with the highest estimated suicide rate in the world with 44.3 suicides per 100,000 inhabitants (p. 20), compared with the average global rate of 11.4 per 100 000 (p.13). Data from the study also showed that there were 946 suicides between 2003 and 2007 (p. 16), a mean of 189 deaths per year. However, 673 persons died as a result of suicide in the three years 2010 to 2012 (p.16), a mean of 224 deaths per year. Additionally, Guyana's Ministry of Public Health Statistics Unit (personal communication, 2017) showed that in the years 2012 and 2014, a total of 646 persons attempted suicide. Figures 7 through 9 show the number of Indo-Guyanese males and females suicidality ratios for the 2010 through 2016.

> WHO (2014) Global Suicide Report recorded Guyana as the country with the highest estimated suicide rate in the world with 44.3 suicides per 100,000 inhabitants.

> Guyana's Ministry of Public Health Statistics Unit (personal communication, 2017) showed that in the years 2012 and 2014, a total of 646 persons attempted suicide.

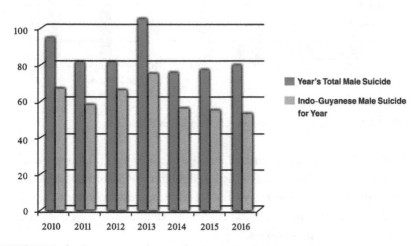

FIGURE 7. Indo-Guyanese male suicides 2010–2016

INDO-GUYANESE FEMALE SUICIDES 2010-2016

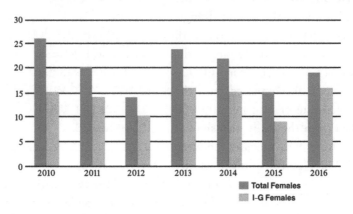

FIGURE 8. Indo-Guyanese female suicides 2010–2016

INDO-GUYANESE MALE vs FEMALE SUICIDES 2010-2016

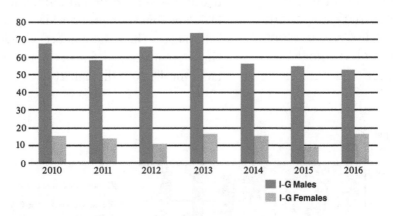

FIGURE 9. Indo-Guyanese male vs female suicides 2010-2016

All the suicide rates are estimated because of the level of underreporting that exists for suicide data. These statistics highlight the problem of regional suicide and suicide attempts among Indo-Guyanese and helped me to determine the five regions with the highest suicidality (Figure 3 above), from which I chose the sample participants.

Suicides and suicide attempts may be individual acts. However, the consequences affect others including family, friends and the community.

Family, Community and Social Influences

Suicide does not affect only the individual concerned but presents a major societal issue, which has an impact on families, communities, and potentially, the identity of a nation. Sociologist Emile Durkheim (1951) theorized that suicide rates increase rapidly as a symptom of the "breakdown of the collective conscience, and of a basic flaw in the social fabric" (p. 7), that is, suicides increase when a society's value system breaks down and "all ameliorative measures must go to the question of the social structure" (p. 7). Kral (1998) used lethality theory to argue that although suicide is ultimately an individual act, it is less an individual act than a product of the collectivity of emotionally charged ideas (pp. 224–225). He highlighted two necessary and sufficient conditions for suicide. The first condition is perturbation, described as "upset, disturbance, agitation, and pain... and acts as motivation when a threshold of tolerance is crossed...but perturbation alone will never lead to or be the cause of suicide" (p. 222). The second condition is lethality, described as "the direct and fatal link to suicide" (p. 223). He argues that all suicide theory is perturbation theory and posits

> Lethality theory is primarily concerned with the idea of suicide, where it comes from, who accepts it, and how forms of this idea are disseminated across and within communities and cultures. Virtually all current suicide theory, from clinical practice to research, is perturbation theory. (p. 223)

My research did not use any specific suicide theory as an initial basis for my exploration. Grounded theory was used to analyze the interview data and to develop theory on the Indo-Guyanese suicide phenomenon, based on the interview data.

Durkheim was one of the first scholars to link suicide with social factors when he described three aetiological types of suicides (pp. 5–6). Firstly, egoistic suicide is the result of person's lack of integration into society, which forces them to live on their own resources (p. 5). Secondly, altruistic suicide is where the person who is "rigorously governed by custom and habit" (p. 6) commits suicide. Thirdly, anomic suicide is the result of lack of regulation by society, in the person's life, in that social and moral norms are unclear or absent (p. 6).

Fushimi (2012) claims that social factors, such as social isolation, influence an individual's suicidal behaviour and, inversely, suicidal behaviour creates anxiety within the society, "seriously affecting families and communities" (p. 69). Social integration, income (economic inequality) and family integration are perceived as indicators of social factors (p. 70). The intensity of the combined forces created by negative social factors (or risk factors) and positive social factors (or protective factors) determine whether the suicide rate increases or decreases.

Keyes (1981) stated that ethnicity is a social construct and not genetically determined; linking humans to the past and is important to the psychological sense of survival (pp. 7–8, 35). As an ethnic group, Indo-Guyanese arrived in Guyana as indentured labourers over 170 years ago, following the abolishment of slavery. Samuel and Wilson (2009) note that emigration was instrumental in breaking up family units because the colonial recruitment process focused on eligible individuals and not on family units (p. 441). For Smith (1959), the breakdown of the Indian caste system, which is the traditional Indian family structure, was due to a plantation life style, shortage of eligible single women, and a lack of landownership. Niehoff and Niehoff (1960) describe how the Indian emigrants were exposed to the colonial and the Afro-Caribbean concepts of family, both of which were alien to their traditional family structure. Ally (1990) states that Indo-Guyanese families were a "very close-knit band of extended lineage, which includes two, three, and often four generations living in close proximity" (para. 4), and that for Indo-Guyanese families, "the general tendency of Indian families and the Indo-Guyanese community generally is to maintain a distinctive and separate identity clearly derived from their attachment to Indian culture" (para. 5). Samuel and Wilson (2009) note that in "the traditional Indian culture, the extended family is considered a better alternative to the nuclear family" (p. 441). Additionally, "The socialization of young girls in patrifocal households, early arranged marriages, low levels of education and the consequent financial dependence on males can explain in part why women strive towards marital stability" (p. 442). Apart from familial, communal and social influences, suicide can also be linked to religious factors next described.

Religious Factors
At the 2012 census in Guyana, Indo-Guyanese Hindus accounted for 24.8% of the religious groups, Christians 64%, and Islam 6.8% (Guyana's Bureau of Statistics, 2012). Samuel and Wilson (2009) state that "traditional religious Hindu women turn to religion and learn to cope with the pressures of marriage life through the teachings of the (Hindu) scriptures" (p. 442).

According to Gearing and Lizardi (2009), suicide is influenced by religion and religion acts as a protective barrier against suicidal behavior (p. 332). Gearing and Lizardi (2009) reviewed "suicide rates and risk and protective factors for suicide across Christianity, Hinduism, Islam, and Judaism" (p. 333). The study shows that "suicide rates and risk and protective factors for suicide vary across religions" (p. 332).

Sisask et al. (2010) found that:

individual-level associations between different dimensions of religiosity and attempting suicide exist. Nevertheless, these associations varied between dimensions of religiosity and across cultures. In particular, subjective religiosity, (considering him/herself to be a religious person) may serve as a protective factor against non-fatal suicidal behaviors in some cultures. (p. 52)

In the Indo-Guyanese context, most persons committing suicide are Hindus. It is therefore helpful to understand the role of religion in the lives of Indo-Guyanese, given that so many Hindus in Guyana as compared to other religions are committing suicide. The Christian Bible states that humanity must not kill. The Sixth Commandment applied to the preservation of all life, which includes one's own life (Exodus 20:13). For Christians, suicide clearly violates the preservation of life. Hindus, on the other hand, believe in reincarnation (Swami Prabhupaba, (n.d.), Chapter 2, verse 27).

Mayer (2010) claims that traditionally, suicides in India are linked to Hindu doctrines of reincarnation and rebirth. The achievement of *moksha* offered freedom from the endless cycle of births, deaths and rebirths (p. 1953). From an Indian historical perspective, according to Radhakrishnan and Andrade (2012):

An understanding of suicide in the Indian context calls for an appreciation of the literary, religious, and cultural ethos of the subcontinent because tradition has rarely permeated the lives of people for as long as it has in India. Ancient Indian texts contain stories of valor in which suicide as a means to avoid shame and disgrace was glorified... The Bhagavad Gita condemns suicide for selfish reasons and posits that such a death cannot have "shraddha," the all-important last rites... Upanishads, the Holy Scriptures, condemn suicide and state that 'he who takes his own life will enter the sunless areas covered by impenetrable darkness after death'. However, the Vedas permit suicide for religious reasons and consider that the best sacrifice was that of one's own life (p. 304).

Psycho-Cultural Processes

Varma (2012) claims that there are two key sociocultural variables that may be related to suicidal behaviour, namely, autonomy and guilt-proneness. He states cultures differ in their dependence and autonomy levels. Traditional, developing Eastern cultures can exemplify dependence chronologically, on "parents, peer groups, spouse and, finally, on one's children" (p. 139), leading to interrelationships where everyone leans on everyone else as opposed to the autonomous self-reliance person who expects everyone to be self-reliant also (p. 139). Additionally, Varma (2012) claims that the autonomy-dependence variable is linked to mental illness, in that when coping fails the underlying anxiety may manifest in psychotic and neurotic symptoms.

An autonomous individual, with his exalted sense of control and mastery over his body, not only assumes greater responsibility over his or her failings, but also assumes the prerogative to do whatever he wants to his body. One of the things that he can do is to kill it....On the other hand, the dependence-prone individual sees cause and effect in a larger context, with the entire milieu participating in it. His failings are not only his, but perhaps reflect what is wrong with the society. Also he is more likely to seek support from his family and friends. (pp. 140–141)

Trotz and Peake (2000) found from their research that the Indians are believed to have striven to retain their cultural uniqueness, by preventing miscegenation (pp. 209–210). This finding aligns with Samuel and Wilson's (2009) findings that Indo-Guyanese are assumed to have retained significant aspects of their cultural heritage. However, they also state that

> limited quantitative empirical data on Indians living in the Caribbean make it difficult to make precise assessments and predictions about the nature of their patterns...Marriage is central to the Indian family and is often not the result of individual efforts but due to combined familial efforts... Divorce is not very common in the traditional Indian culture, but this does not mean that all Indians are very happy in their relationships. Many Indian couples live together even though they do not like each other because they fear the social disapproval of divorce. (pp. 440–442)

Medora, Larson, and Dave (2000) note conformity is valued over self-identity and self-expression. Group identity and cohesiveness is stressed and a conservative and compliant orientation is rewarded (pp. 415–416). It is probable that some Indo-Guyanese have committed suicide in an attempt to avoid staying in unhappy relationships. I wonder if suicide would have been an option if there were a platform for them to share their pain.

Understanding through Phenomenology

'Phenomenology' is a collection and analysis of people's perceptions related to a specific, definable phenomenon... Perception [is] the lived experience, how people relate to a phenomenon, how people understand a phenomenon, and the meaning people give a phenomenon.

According to Burkholder, Cox, and Crawford (2016), 'phenomenology' is "a collection and analysis of people's perceptions related to a specific, definable phenomenon... Perception [is] the lived experience, how people relate to a phenomenon, how people understand a phenomenon, and the meaning people give a phenomenon" (pp. 203–204). "Phenomenology can help you understand the human factors involved in an experience" such as suicide.

To truly listen to another person, it is essential that we are aware of our own biases, our worldview, and the potential impact of our biases on how we interpret what the other person is saying. As suicide attempters subjectively make meaning of their lived experiences, family-member survivors grapple with attempting to understand the reason their loved ones committed suicide.

Psychological Autopsy Interviews

Cassells et al's (2005) psychological autopsy shows that suicide completers often have experienced recent loss, grief, shame, and/or feelings of hopelessness (pp. 53–63). Additionally, according to Harwood et al. (2002), suicide survivors can be left with "a mixture of loss, hopelessness, grief, and shame" (pp. 185–194).

An example psychological autopsy interview carried out by Cheng et al. (2000) highlighted that psychological autopsy studies among suicide completers have consistently shown "a high prevalence of mental disorders in people who have committed suicide in both Eastern and Western countries… The most common types of disorder have been depressive illness and alcoholism" (p. 360). The psychological autopsy interviews were conducted by a psychiatrist and two psychologists who interviewed key informants of the suicides, as well as a control group. "The interview was designed to assess mental, personality and physical disorders, family history, stressful life events, and socio-demographic data" (p. 361). Information on the family tree, and key persons familiar with the suicides and controls were obtained to find as many potential interviewees as possible (pp. 360-361).

The findings of Cheng et al. (2000) in some way contrast with Crichton-Miller's view, which points out that it is not the illness but the fear of having the illness that drives a person to suicide (p. 240). Similar to Cheng and colleagues, suicide psychological autopsy studies by Cavanagh et al. (2003) also found that mental disorder was the leading variable associated with suicide and suggested that "further studies should focus on specific disorders and psychosocial factors" (p. 395). They pointed out that the major obstacle to truly understanding suicide is that although the victim cannot be

Better understanding of the suicide may be gained from looking at the family-member survivor's perspective, at what the survivor's life was like, post-suicide.

interviewed but it helped to interview the closest relatives, and to review appropriate evidence, such as hospital case notes, in order to get to know the deceased (p. 395). The example from Cheng et al. of psychological autopsy has important features for developing psychological autopsy interviews (p. 361), but better understanding of the suicide may be gained from looking at the family-member survivor's perspective, at what the survivor's life was like, post-suicide. I believe that grounded theory was an apt research methodology for constructing meaning from all the participants' stories.

Constructing a Sociological Reality

According to Charmaz (1990):

> the grounded theory method itself offers a way of constructing sociological reality; using the method fosters developing analytic and conceptual constructions of the data. In their sociological constructions, grounded theorists aim to create theoretical categories from the data and then analyze relationships between key categories. In short, the researcher constructs theory from the data. By starting with data from the lived experience of the research participants, the researcher can, from the beginning, attend to how they construct their worlds. That lived experience shapes the researcher's approach to data collection and analysis. (p. 1162)

Kral stated "a deeper understanding of suicide will be realized through theory incorporating the dialectic of person and culture" (p. 221). Kral believes "the time is right to use 'anthropological imagination' in suicidology and that (researchers) must begin to examine the cultural narratives of suicide and their impact on individuals and groups" (p. 230). The aim is "to foster the development of a conceptual language with important consequences for research, practice, and prevention." I believe that a person-centered approach in interacting with persons with suicidal ideation helps to provide understanding on how they symbolically interact with others in their environment.

Symbolic Interactionism

Blumer (1969) states symbolic interactionism rests on three premises.

Firstly:

> human beings act toward things on the basis of the meanings that the things have for them... to ignore the meaning of the things towards which people act is to falsify the behavior under study and to bypass the meaning in favor of factors alleged to produce the behavior is seen as a grievous neglect of the role of meaning in the formation of behavior. (pp. 2, 3)

Secondly:

> the meaning of such things is derived from, or arises out of, the social interaction that one has with one's fellows... the meaning of a thing for a person grows out of the ways in which other persons act toward the person with regard to the thing. Their actions operate to define the thing for the person. Thus, symbolic interactionism sees meanings as social products, as creations that are formed in and through the defining activities of people as they interact. (pp. 2, 4)

Thirdly:

> these meanings are handled in, and modified through, an interpretative process used by the person in dealing with the things he encounters...interpretation should not be regarded as a mere automatic application of established meanings but as a formative process in which meanings are used and revised as instruments for the guidance and formation of action. (pp. 2, 5)

The study concludes that meanings are therefore lodged respectively in the thing, in the psyche and in social action, and are "handled flexibly by the actor in the course of forming his action" (pp. 5-6).

Symbolic interactionism is compatible with grounded theory, and I believe it is a helpful knowledge-base when researching suicides, in terms of recognizing why people behave the way they do and how they make meaning of their lived experiences.

Aldiabat and Le Navenec (2011) claim that:

> Symbolic Interactionism provides a guiding framework to collect data about the meaning of a particular type of behaviour and the contextual sources of such meanings, and how they change in and through social and physical time and space; and... Grounded Theory methodology affords a systematic approach to generate a theory that illuminates human behaviour as a social process among actors in their interactional context. (p. 1068)

According to LaRossa and Reitzes (2009), symbolic interactionism:

> focuses on the connection between symbols (i.e., shared meanings) and interactions (i.e., verbal and nonverbal actions and communications). It essentially is a frame of reference for understanding how humans, in concert with one another, create symbolic worlds and how these worlds, in turn, shape human behavior. (pp. 135–136)

Exploring how people behave in their own contexts provides understanding when researching behaviour in relation to the meanings people place on social conditions and influences. Aldiabac and Le Navenec (2011) argue that:

> human beings respond to a particular situation through how they define that situation, rather than how the situation is objectively presented to them. Therefore, an understanding about how humans define the situation can assist us to more fully comprehend why they behave as they do in the situation. (p. 1067)

Meaning is formed in the context of social interaction. As human beings interact socially with each other, meaning is co-constructed and, depending on individual perspective, the result is either a positive or negative relationship outcome or experience. According to Blumer (1969), through social interactions, human beings become aware of what others are doing or about what they are willing to do. As a result, through a process referred to as 'joint action', they modify their behaviours based on the behaviours of others with whom they interact (p. 17).

'Self' is a social construct because, according to Aldiabac and Le Navenec

(2011), "human beings can constantly change themselves through their interaction with others" (p. 1076). LaRossa and Reitzes state that healthy self-concepts are developed through social interaction with others and "provide an important motive for behavior" (p. 144). According to Aldiabac and Le Navenec:

> Sometimes humans evaluate themselves, plan for future action, and punish or reward themselves. Based on this internal interaction, humans act in relation to others as well as toward themselves. In other words, if one is to understand human interaction/ interactions of others, one must first gain an understanding of the meaning of the self-concept. (p. 1065)

> Through social interactions, human beings become aware of what others are doing or about what they are willing to do. As a result, through a process referred to as 'joint action', they modify their behaviours based on the behaviours of others with whom they interact.

Gecas (1982) states that the self-concept is "the concept the individual has of himself as a physical, social, spiritual or moral being" (p. 3). In his discussion on the self-concept theory, Purkey (1988) states:

> Because of previous experiences and present perceptions, individuals may perceive themselves in ways different from the ways others see them.
> – Individuals perceive different aspects of themselves at different times with varying degrees of clarity. Therefore, inner focusing is a valuable tool for counselling.
> – Any experience which is inconsistent with one's self-concept may be perceived as a threat, and the more of these experiences there are, the more rigidly self-concept is organized to maintain and protect itself. When a person is unable to get rid of perceived inconsistencies, emotional problems arise.
> – Faulty thinking patterns, such as dichotomous reasoning (dividing everything in terms of opposites or extremes) or overgeneralizing (making sweeping conclusions based on little information) create negative interpretations of oneself. (paras. 17–19)

Inconsistencies of self-concept and dichotomous reasoning, for example, pose a number of challenges in social relationships and can lead to suicide. Grounded theory is a valuable tool in providing understanding of what participants perceive as reality based on their self-concepts.

Constructing Reality

In the process of gaining meaning from interview data, Charmaz (1990) claims that the direction of grounded theory interviews sets the tone in order to seek information, feeling, and reflection. The perspective taken will inform the development of the schedule including the questions asked, the nature of the relationship, and the ways in which questions are delivered (p. 1167).

Wimpenny and Gass (2000) note the grounded theory interview will be less open and more structured in style (p. 1490). O'Reilly and Kiyimba (2015) note that a phenomenologist is most likely to bracket off personal involvement in the interview to focus on eliciting narratives about the lived experiences of the participants (p. 80).

Summary

In an attempt to identify the factors that may lead to Indo-Guyanese suicide, which are often underreported, I have presented numerous literary views in this chapter. I have proffered reasons why people commit suicide and described the psychology and nature of suicide, including mental and emotional factors. I have also discussed the value of grounded theory in providing a platform for making meaning of participants' realities. Exploring the basic tenets of symbolic interactionism provided understanding of self, self-concept and how humans interact with each other. In the next chapter, I will look at some biblical and theological principles in relation to suicide.

REFERENCE LIST

Aldiabat, K. M. and Le Navenec, C. L. (2011). Philosophical roots of classical grounded theory: Its foundations in symbolic interactionism. *The Qualitative Report*, 16(4), 1063.

Ally, B. (1990). Indo-Caribbean life in Guyana and Toronto: A comparative survey. Retrieved from http://archives.commissiondesetudiants.ca/magic/mt25.html

Barbour, J. D. (1994). Suicide, tragedy, and theology in "Sophie's Choice" and Gustafson's theocentric ethics. *Literature and Theology*, 8(1), 80–93.

Bertolote, J. M. and Fleischmann, A. (2002). A global perspective in the epidemiology of suicide. *Suicidologi*, 7(2), 6–8.

Blumer, H. (1969). *Symbolic Interaction: Perspective and Method*. New Jersey: Englewood Cliffs.

Burkholder, G. J., Cox, K. and Crawford, L. (eds.) (2016). *The Scholar-Practitioner's Guide to Research Design*. Baltimore, MD: Laureate Publishing. Vitalbook file.

Caribbean360. Second suicide in two months at Guyana's Kaieteur Falls. (2015, November 23). Retrieved from http://www.caribbean360.com/news/second-suicide-in-two-months-at-guyanas-kaieteur-falls

Cassells, C., Paterson, B., Dowding, D. and Morrison, R. (2005). Long-and short-term risk factors in the prediction of inpatient suicide: A review of the literature. *Crisis*, 26(2), 53-63.

Cavanagh, J. T., Carson, A. J., Sharpe, M. and Lawrie, S. M. (2003). Psychological autopsy studies of suicide: a systematic review. *Psychological Medicine*, 33(3), 395-405.

Charmaz, K. (1990). 'Discovering' chronic illness: Using grounded theory. *Social Science & Medicine*, 30(11), 1161–1172.

Cheng, A. T., Chen, T. H., Chen, C. C. and Jenkins, R. (2000). Psychosocial and psychiatric risk factors for suicide. *The British Journal of Psychiatry*, 177(4), 360–365.

Cornette, M. M., Mathias, C.W., Marsh, D. M., DeRoon-Cassini, T. A. and Dougherty, D. M. (2012). Cognition and Suicide. In *Suicide from a Global Perspective: Psychosocial Approaches*. (pp. 1–10). New York: Nova Science Publishers, Inc.

Crocker, J. and Major, B. (1989). Social stigma and self-esteem: The self-protective properties of stigma. *Psychological Review*, 96(4), 608-630.

Crichton-Miller, H. (1931). The psychology of suicide. *British Medical Journal*, 2(3683), 239–241.

De Groot, M. and Kollen, B. J. (2013). Course of bereavement over 8-10 years in first degree relatives and spouses of people who committed suicide: longitudinal community based cohort study. *BMJ*, 347, f5519.

Doka, K. J. (ed.) (2014). *Living with grief: After sudden loss suicide, homicide, accident, heart attack, stroke*. Oxford: Taylor & Francis.

Durkheim, E. (1951). *Suicide: A study in sociology* (JA Spaulding & G. Simpson, trans.). Glencoe, IL: Free Press. (*Original work published 1897*).

Fraser, J. M. (2017, March 21). Guyana's suicide rate is the highest in the world. Kaieteur News. Retrieved from https://www.kaieteurnewsonline. com/2017/03/21/guyanas-suicide-rate-is-the-highest-in-the-world/

Fushimi, M. (2012). Sociological Perspectives on Suicide. In *Suicide from a Global Perspective: Psychosocial Approaches*. (pp. 69–74). New York: Nova Science.

Gearing, R. E. and Lizardi, D. (2009). Religion and suicide. *Journal of Religion and Health*, 48(3), 332–341.

Gecas, V. (1982). The self-concept. *Annual Review of Sociology*, 8(1), 1–33.

Guyana. Bureau of Statistics. (2012). 2012 Population and Housing Census. Retrieved from https://www.statisticsguyana.gov.gy/census.html Final_2012_ Census_Compendium2.pdf

Guyana. Ministry of Public Health. (2014). *National Suicide Prevention Plan: A National Suicide Prevention Strategy for Guyana (2015-2020)* [Brochure]. Guyana: Pan American Health Organization.

Harwood, D., Hawton, K., Hope, T. and Jacoby, R. (2002). The grief experiences and needs of bereaved relatives and friends of older people dying through suicide: a descriptive and case-control study. *Journal of Affective Disorders*, 72(2), 185–194.

Hutchinson, G., Daisley, H., Simmons, V., & Gordon, A. N. (1991). Suicide by poisoning. *The West Indian Medical Journal*, 40(2), 69–73.

Jordan, J. R. (2015). Grief after suicide: The evolution of suicide postvention. In *Death, dying and bereavement: Contemporary perspectives, institutions and practices*, (pp. 349–362). New York, NY: Springer.

Jordan, J. R. and McIntosh, J. L. (eds.) (2011). *Grief after suicide: Understanding the consequences and caring for the survivors*. England: Routledge.

Katz, C., Bolton, J. and Sareen, J. (2016). The prevalence rates of suicide are likely underestimated worldwide: why it matters. *Social Psychiatry and Psychiatric Epidemiology*, 51(1), 125-127.

Keyes, C. F. (1981). The dialectics of ethnic change. *Ethnic change*, 30.

Kral, M. J. (1998). Suicide and the internalization of culture: Three questions. *Transcultural Psychiatry*, 35(2), 221–233.

LaRossa, R. and Reitzes, D. C. (2009). Symbolic interactionism and family studies. In *Sourcebook of Family Theories and Methods* (pp. 135–166). New York: Springer Science & Business Media, Inc.

Maharajh, H. D. and Abdool, P. S. (2005). Cultural aspects of suicide. *The Scientific World Journal*, 5, 736–746.

Mayer, P. (2010). *Suicide and Society in India*. England: Routledge.

Medora, N., Larson, J. and Dave, P. (2000). East-Indian college student's perceptions of family strengths. Retrieved from http://www.jstor.org/stable/41603710

McKenzie, K., Serfaty, M. and Crawford, M. (2003). Suicide in ethnic minority groups. *British Journal of Psychiatry*, 183, 100–101.

Mościcki, E. K. (2001). Epidemiology of completed and attempted suicide: toward a framework for prevention. *Clinical Neuroscience Research*, 1(5), 310–323.

Niehoff, A. H. and Niehoff, J. (1960). *East Indians in the West Indies (No. 6)*. Milwaukee, WI: Milwaukee Public Museum.

Nock, M. K., Borges, G., Bromet, E. J., Cha, C. B., Kessler, R. C. and Lee, S. (2008). Suicide and suicidal behavior. *Epidemiologic reviews*, 30(1), 133–154.

Nolen-Hoeksema, S. (1991). Responses to depression and their effects on the duration of depressive episodes. *Journal of Abnormal Psychology*, 100(4), 569.

O'Reilly, M. and Kiyimba, N. (2015). *Advanced Qualitative Research: A Guide to Using Theory*. California: Sage.

Overholser, J. C., Adams, D. M., Lehnert, K. L. and Brinkman, D. C. (1995). Self-esteem deficits and suicidal tendencies among adolescents. *Journal of the American Academy of Child & Adolescent Psychiatry*, 34(7), 919–928.

Purkey, W. W. (1988). An Overview of Self-Concept Theory for Counselors. Highlights: An ERIC/CAPS Digest. Retrieved from http://ericae.net/edo/ed304630.htm

Radhakrishnan, R., & Andrade, C. (2012). Suicide: an Indian perspective. *Indian Journal of Psychiatry*, 54(4), 304–319.

Samuel, P. S. and Wilson, L. C. (2009). Structural arrangements of Indo-Guyanese family: An assessment of the assimilation hypothesis. *Journal of Comparative Family Studies*, 40(3), 439–454.

Scocco, P. and Toffol, E. (2012). Loss, Hopelessness and Suicide. In *Suicide from a global perspective: psychosocial approaches*. (pp. 11–17). New York: Nova Science.

Sharma, S. D., & Gopalakrishna, R. (1978). Suicide – A retrospective study in a culturally distinct community in India. *International Journal of Social Psychiatry*, 24(1), 13–18.

Shneidman, E. S. (1993). Commentary: Suicide as psychache. *The Journal of Nervous and Mental disease*, 181(3), 145147.

Sisask, M., Värnik, A., Kolves, K., Bertolote, J. M., Bolhari, J., Botega, N.J., Fleischmann, A., Vijayakumar, L. and Wasserman, D. (2010). Is religiosity a protective factor against attempted suicide: a cross-cultural case-control study. *Archives of Suicide Research*, 14(1), 44–55.

Smith, R. T. (1959). Some social characteristics of Indian immigrants to British Guiana. Population Studies, 13(1), 34-39.

Spokas, M., Wenzel, A., Brown, G. K. and Beck, A. T. (2012). Characteristics of individuals who make impulsive suicide attempts. *Journal of affective disorders*, 136(3), 1121–1125.

Swami Prabhupada, B. S. S. (n.d.). Srimad Bhagavad-Gita and Reincarnation. Retrieved from http://www.bhagavad-gita.org/Articles/gita-reincarnation.html

Tøllefsen, I. M., Hem, E. and Ekeberg, Ø. (2012). The reliability of suicide statistics: a systematic review. *BMC psychiatry*, *12*(1), 9.

Trotz, D. A. and Peake, L. (2000). Work, family, and organising: an overview of the emergence of the economic, social and political roles of women in British Guiana. *Social and Economic Studies*, 49(4), 189–222.

Van Orden, K. A., Witte, T. K., Cukrowicz, K. C., Braithwaite, S. R., Selby, E. A. and Joiner Jr, T. E. (2010). The interpersonal theory of suicide. *Psychological Review*, 117(2), 575.

Varma, V. K. (2012). Cultural Psychodynamics and Suicidal Behavior. In *Suicide from a Global Perspective: Psychosocial Approaches*. (pp. 137-144). New York: Nova Science.

Wertheimer, A. (2013). *A Special Scar: The experiences of people bereaved by suicide*. England: Routledge.

Wimpenny, P. and Gass, J. (2000). Interviewing in phenomenology and grounded theory: is there a difference? *Journal of Advanced Nursing*, 31(6), 1485–1492.

World Health Organization. (2000). *Preventing suicide: A resource for media professionals* [Brochure]. World Health Organization.

World Health Organization. (2014). *Preventing suicide: A global imperative* [Brochure]. World Health Organization.

World Health Organization. (2018). World Health Statistics data visualizations dashboard. Retrieved from http://apps.who.int/gho/data/node.sdg.3-4-viz-2?lang=en

PART 3
THEOLOGICAL PERSPECTIVES

CHAPTER 5

BIBLICAL AND THEOLOGICAL FOUNDATIONS

Religious commitment, measured in terms of a few core beliefs and
practices, many be a powerful counteragent against suicide. That is,
the mere number of shared beliefs and practices is not important.
Rather, despite what Durkheim said to the contrary, the content of
religion is important.
(Stack, 1983)

Introduction

I question if one can make biblical or theological sense of the suicide of
a person, Christian or non-Christian, who has been experiencing intense
pain and suffering. This chapter provides the biblical and theological basis
for understanding how suicide is perceived from a Christian perspective.
Using biblical examples and key theological doctrines, this chapter focuses
on the tragedy of suicide by looking at, for example, human suffering and
the Sovereignty of God. The chapter looks at the Church's response to suicide
and how the peace Jesus offers is instrumental in alleviating the pain that
leads to suicide ideation and suicide. There is understanding that most of the
Indo-Guyanese who commit or attempt suicide are Hindus and will not all
be fully conversant with Christian theology as discussed in this chapter.

Biblical Perspective on Suicide

Suicide, as considered in this study, is a voluntary and intentional desire for
self destruction. In its simplest form, suicide is the taking one's life on purpose. Suicide is not a new phenomenon. The word *suicide* does not appear in
the Bible; however, there are biblical records of at least seven cases of known

suicides. They include Judas (Matthew 2:5), who hanged himself after he betrayed Jesus; Samson (Judges 16:25–31), who killed himself while killing a large number of Philistines in revenge for causing him much pain and the loss of his freedom; King Saul, after being severely wounded, (1 Samuel 31:4), in hopelessness and the dread of being tortured by the Philistines, committed suicide; King Saul's armour-bearer (1 Samuel 31:5), who being overwhelmed at King Saul's suicide, killed himself; Ahithophel (2 Samuel 17:23) filled with disappointment at the rejection of his advice, hanged himself; and Zimri (I King 16:18–19), who in an act of revenge, burnt down the palace in which he reigned for only seven days, while he was in it, thereby killing himself.

According to Barraclough (1992), the Bible treats these biblical suicides in a factual way and not as wrong or shameful (p. 64). However, as the Israelites journeyed from Egypt to the Promised Land of Canaan, God gave strict instructions through the Ten Commandments to their leader, Moses. The Israelites were expected to obey the instructions in order to live in a close and acceptable relationship with God. The Sixth Commandment in Exodus 20:13, "You shall not murder" is a key Scripture concerning the taking of life.

Cook (2014) noted that in Hebrew Scripture, suicide is implicitly condemned in the Sixth Commandment, and both Jewish and Christian commentators have generally seen suicide to be forbidden by this commandment (p. 4). Gill (2006) highlighted that fourth century theologian and philosopher, Augustine of Hippo, argued that "a man is not allowed to kill himself, since the text 'Thou shall not kill' has no addition and it must be taken that there is no exception, not even the one to whom the command is addressed" (p. 352). According to Jacobs (1995), Jewish law does not consider the Sixth Commandment as applying to suicide, but it does value the preservation of human life above all else, and thus effectively condemns suicide (p. 501).

I wondered how a Christian's faith related to suicide. According to Honderich (2005), philosophical controversy has included paternalism in suicide intervention (p. 902). Honderich (2005) states paternalism is:

> The power and authority one person or institution exercises over another to confer benefits or prevent harm for the latter regardless of the latter's informed consent. Paternalism is thus a threat to autonomy as well as to liberty and privacy. On any normative theory, however, paternalism is desirable toward young children, the mentally ill, and others similarly situated. (p. 684)

And:

> If individuals have a *right* to commit suicide, then others appear to have a correlative obligation not to intervene to prevent the suicide. Yet we often do intervene, either by reporting a suicide threat or preventing a suicide attempt....

> No one doubts that we should intervene to prevent suicide by incompetent persons. But if we accept an unrestricted, free choice principle, the imprudent but competent suicide who would want to live under more favourable circumstances could not legitimately be prevented from committing suicide (p. 902).

Honderich concludes that both the "law and philosophy continue to struggle with issues about the extent to which paternalism is justified in such cases, if it is" (p. 902).

Honderich's (2005) logic briefly touches on the free-will doctrine which a Christian believes that God has granted to each individual. However, like many, I question if this free-will choice extends to humans taking their own lives, and if there is a place for responsibility in the preservation of life, and the paternalism of suicide intervention.

Apostle Paul taught the Galatian Christians, "You, my brothers and sisters, were called to be free. But do not use your freedom to indulge the flesh; rather, serve one another humbly in love" (Galatians 5:13). Freedom that Christians receive through Christ should not be seen as an opportunity to do whatever the carnal flesh wants to do, but, instead, freedom is intended to serve others in love. Submission to works of the flesh can create intense pain which can lead to suicide. This scenario is evidenced when Judas was filled with remorse over his betrayal of Jesus and hanged himself (Matthew 27:3-5). On the other hand, the Bible indicates that in all of Job's intense suffering, he chose not to see it as an opportunity to sin but instead to proclaim his faith in God. Job said "Though he slay me, yet will I hope in him" (Job 13:15a). Job did not have the Holy Spirit residing in him as born-again Christians do, but Job had faith and hope in the Sovereignty and omnipotence of God.

The book of Job shows the inherent sinful nature of humans from the verse "Yet man is born to trouble as surely as sparks fly upward" (Job 5:7); and the limitation of human understanding from Job 11:7–9 which states:

Can you fathom the mysteries of God? Can you probe the limits of the Almighty? They are higher than the heavens above—what can you do? They are deeper than the depths below—what can you know? Their measure is longer than the earth and wider than the sea.

> People who are hurting often tend to find an object to place the blame for their hurt.

The book of Job also explores accusations of God being unjust.

It is all the same; that is why I say, He destroys both the blameless and the wicked. When a scourge brings sudden death, he mocks the despair of the innocent. When a land falls into the hands of the wicked, he blindfolds its judges. If it is not he, then who is it? (9:22–24)

People who are hurting often tend to find an object to place the blame for their hurt. Job accuses God of being unjust because he sees God as destroying both the blameless and the wicked (9:22) and of blindfolding earthly judges (9:24). Barbour (1994) states:

An untimely death by suicide may make us angry not only at the person who chooses to die, and at the society in which she lives, but at God. Such a death may make us ask the classical questions about whether God lacks the power or the goodness to have helped the individual find a way to carry on. We may wonder whether the despairing suicide could ever be reconciled with God, and how God's grace can reach a person who performs what many Christians have described as an unforgiveable sin, the rejection of God's gift of life. (pp. 82–83)

Koch (2005) states that suicide is not explicitly condemned nor approved in Judeo-Christian Scripture, and noted that the Bible considers human life as a divine gift. Those suffering from suicidal ideation must be treated with respect and support should be offered (p. 167).

The book of Job describes the relationship humans need to have with God, in spite of any suffering being experienced, because without God's intervention, the devil is free to do whatever he desires in people's lives. God is

Past and Current Perspectives on Suicide

In comparing the suicide rates within Catholicism and Protestantism, Durkheim (1951) argued that higher social integration and regulation in Catholicism encouraged lower suicide rates (p. 5). Stark, Doyle, and Rushing (1983) challenged Durkheim's theory by claiming that although religion matters because religious commitment offers a protective effect, it is not only related to the Catholics but to all religions (p.126). Stack and Wasserman (1992) also challenged Durkheim's theory with their religious network theory, claiming that since Durkheim's work on religious integration/affiliation,

sociocultural trends, secularization, ecumenicalism, and evangelical revival have altered the relationship between religion and society. As a consequence, some Protestant denominations are now associated with relatively high suicide rates, while other Protestant denominations are associated with relatively low rates. (p. 458)

According to Mowat, Swinton, Stark, and Mowat (2013), "Most mainstream religious groups are likely to provide some protection against suicide. This protection is probably greatest when congregations have the greatest interaction with one another, can respond in a crisis, and counsel against suicide" (p. 1). They further added that:

Faith communities can provide a counter-cultural view of the world and an alternative set of values and criteria for being human and living humanly. As such they are in a position to reframe the expectations and value systems of adherents. A key potential for faith communities is to redefine the idea of progress. (p. 2)

Finally they claim that:

Ministers felt that the completed suicide act was explainable in terms of trying to find peace and of ceasing to hurt others. They also felt that the Church did not give a strong lead, and that the disconnection was due to lack of faith. No faith in anything other than oneself, or a misinterpretation of theology based on myth and prejudice, made people very vulnerable. (p. 3)

Gearing and Lizardi (2009) state that "The view of suicide as a sin dominates current Christian attitudes across the various denominations (e.g., Catholics, Baptists, and Protestants)" (p. 334). However, according to *Libreria Editrice Vaticana* (2003), individuals have to be mentally competent to understand that the act in which they partake is a sin. "Grave psychological disturbances, anguish, or grave fear of hardship, suffering, or torture can diminish the responsibility of the one committing suicide" (para. 2282). "Thus, if one considers suicide an act of the mentally ill, it cannot simultaneously be viewed a sin" (Gearing and Lizardi, p. 334) and only God as the judge can determine the outcome of a person's death (ibid.).

Factors Contributing to Suicide within the Church

I believe that the Church has had its own challenges regarding suicide, which for some onlookers may make a moral response from it questionable. McKenzie, Baker, and Lee (2012) reported on the number of suicides that had occurred because of sexual abuse of young men by named Catholic priests. The report said, "It appears that up to 34 males have suicided... all appear to relate to their contact with [alleged perpetrators' names withheld]....it would appear that an investigation would uncover many more deaths as a consequence of clergy abuse" (p. 1). The report was just one of many reports that occurred globally within the last decade, and it may make some wonder why the Church should be listened to as an authority in morality and social justice.

According to Waddell (personal communication, 2017), "It can be quite a traumatic experience for adults when trust in the spiritual leaders, who are responsible for their spiritual and moral well-being, has been breached, often leading to damaged faith and even suicide." The victim's nuclear family is often affected because as Waddell states, "You cannot sin in isolation... your action will impact and affect others." I believe that, where lacking, confidence in the Church and in church leaders can be restored but only when there is a major public relations exercise in which the Church becomes very transparent in its activity of investigating each charge made

> It can be quite a traumatic experience for adults when trust in the spiritual leaders, who are responsible for their spiritual and moral well-being, has been breached, often leading to damaged faith and even suicide.

against those accused, without prejudice, publicly repenting, returning to biblical teaching in holiness, and providing professional counselling for the perpetrators. Further, Waddell added that through

> biblical teaching, the community in general and the abused can find moral guidance, solace, and comfort in the inspired Word of God based on 2 Timothy 3:16, which says 'All Scripture is God-breathed and is useful for teaching, rebuking, correcting and training in righteousness.

I believe that it is important for the Church to strongly refocus on Jesus' ministry and comprehensively review the Church's current position against the biblical tenets and the key leadership styles portrayed by Jesus, which included Servant Leadership and Shalom Leadership. Jesus came to earth to humbly serve His creation. Jesus left His Heavenly location in order to show His creation how to live pleasing to God. For church leaders to remain in their positions, they must be totally committed to living the exemplar life of Jesus in the community in which they are called to serve. There needs to be better and regular checks, including mental functionality checks, on church leaders for their benefit as well as those they serve.

Leclaire (2013) states that pastors are not exempt from committing suicide (paras. 1–3). The reasons cited include depression, which many pastors do not accept as a mental illness, low pay, burnout and spirituality (paras. 5-7). According to London and Wiseman (2003):

> Pastors have an incredibly significant and difficult job. (He) is that person we know as the professional minister – a human being like the rest of us, who increasingly finds himself working against a legion of obstacles, unrealistic expectations, and stresses and strains unique to his position in the world. (p. 9)

Given the discussions in this section, the Church has a significant role to play in obeying both the Great Commission and the Great Commandment if there is to be God's shalom.

The Concept of Shalom as Related to Suicide

"Shalom," the Hebrew word for *"peace,"* which BGU (2017) describes in its Shalom leadership perspective as "well-being, abundance, and wholeness of the community as well as individuals." Shalom leadership style is reconciliatory in its objective. The study by Mowat et al. (2013) on the role of the Church in relation to suicide found that "Ministers felt that the completed suicide act was explainable in terms of trying to find peace and of ceasing to hurt others" (p. 3).

Many writers and clinicians have made a link to depression and suicide. WHO (n.d.) defines *depression* as "a common mental disorder, characterized by sadness, loss of interest or pleasure, feelings of guilt or low self-worth, disturbed sleep or appetite, feelings of tiredness, and poor concentration."

> "Shalom," the Hebrew word for "peace," which BGU (2017) describes in its Shalom leadership perspective as "well-being, abundance, and wholeness of the community as well as individuals."

Depression and shalom are on opposite sides of the spectrum. Many of King David's Psalms are replete with his struggles with depression. In Psalm 6 to the Chief Musician as a penitent song, David is agonized, depressed, and discouraged as he feels God's chastisement as a result of sin. David pens in verse 6 "I am worn out with grief; every night my bed is damp from my weeping; my pillow is soaked with tears" (GNT). In the Psalm of transition, Psalm 13 to the Chief Musician, David is in despair, feeling lonely and thinking God has forgotten him; he experiences daily sorrow so severe to the point of asking God, in verse 4, not to let him die from his grief. In Psalm 38:6, 8 full of grief from his sins and affliction, David wrote "I am bowed down

> Many writers and clinicians have made a link to depression and suicide. WHO (n.d.) defines depression as "a common mental disorder, characterized by sadness, loss of interest or pleasure, feelings of guilt or low self-worth, disturbed sleep or appetite, feelings of tiredness, and poor concentration."

Severe grief can lead to depression.

and brought very low; all day long I go about mourning... I am feeble and utterly crushed; I groan in anguish of heart." King David's depression is experienced by both believers and non-believers alike. David turned to God as a cure for his depression, repented where needed, and felt the restoration of shalom.

Severe grief can lead to depression. Mourning the loss of a suicide victim is often complex and lengthier than other losses, according to Brown (1999). Family-member survivors and friends of the deceased are left with endless unanswered questions as well as stigma, guilt, shame, and rejection. For Christians, finding peace in a tragic situation comes from knowing that God is not responsible for death, but the sin that has tainted all of humanity results in death. It may be impossible to find answers to the death, but it is valuable to know that just as the heart of the survivors break so does God's heart, for Christians and non-Christians (pp. 83, 103).

Apostle Paul, in 2 Corinthians 12:7–9, spoke about a "thorn in his flesh" that he had asked God to remove three times, but God had told him that His grace was sufficient for him. Some theologians believe Apostle Paul was suffering from depression (Pollock, 2012, p. 79; MacArthur, 2010, pp. 85–86). Paul's missionary experience and affliction in Asia made him describe life in 2 Corinthians 1:8-9a; 4:8-10a as utterly burdened, struck down, perplexed and seemingly in a death

Mood disorders, especially depressive disorders are prevalent, hard to treat, and cause considerable morbidity.

sentence. Whatever the suffering, Paul's peace, as shown by his situational responses, came from his relationship with the true and living God.

Hashmi, Butt, and Umair (2013) note that mood disorders, especially depressive disorders are prevalent, hard to treat, and cause considerable morbidity. They describe depression as a "complex illness that is associated with substantial disability and reduced quality of life for the person with depression, as well as a significant social burden" (p. 899). Phipps (1985) noted that in 1980, the New York-based organization Concern for Dying convened a group of psychiatrists, philosophers, and theologians who prepared a statement on suicide for the terminally ill.

Historically, suicide has been judged as 'sinful' by organized religion...
We do not dispute the contention that the majority of suicides represent a rejection of the 'gift of life' and, as such, are evidence of severe
emotional distress. We believe, however, that a person with a progres-
sive terminal disease faces a unique situation – one which calls for a
new look at traditional assumptions about the motivation for choosing suicide. In our view, this choice might be found to be reasoned,
appropriate, altruistic, sacrificial, and loving. We can imagine that an
individual faced with debilitating, irreversible illness, who would have
to endure intractable pain, mutilating surgery, or demeaning treat-
ments – with added concern for the burden being placed on family
and friends – might conclude that suicide was a reasonable, even gen-
erous, resolution to a process already moving inexorably toward death.
(para. 19)

I believe that the gift of life is a precious gift and not intended by God to be
dispensed with, either recklessly nor prematurely, regardless of the reason.
I believe that a loving God never gives believers more than they are able
to cope with, and who knows God's mind for those persons suffering any
illness, including terminal illness. I also believe that God does not desire
His creation to suffer. However, the enemy, Satan, sets out to destroy the life
which God through Jesus intends for believers to enjoy in abundance. As
Jesus said, "The thief comes only to steal and kill and destroy; I have come
that they may have life, and have it to the full" (John 10:10).

The question may be asked 'What happens to sufferers of depression, such
as the Indo-Guyanese Hindus, who do not have the God of King David
and Apostle Paul to turn to?' I believe that there is one sure way for shalom
to replace suicidal behaviour, and that is through a relationship similar to
what God desired to have with the early Israelites. For non-believers, this
kind of relationship does not exist, and, as such, the believer is compelled
to action through the Great Commission (Matthew 28:18–20) and Great
Commandment (Matthew 22:36–40). How this action is worked out
depends on the believer's giftedness, calling, and purpose in life.

Summary

In this chapter, I have discussed biblical examples of suicide and theological principles on the Church's response to suicide. I have looked at past and present perspectives on suicides and areas in which the Church has failed its congregants, and, to some extent, its leadership. I have discussed how Hindus' beliefs in reincarnation can lead to hopelessness and how God's shalom through the examples of Jesus can help to mitigate suicides, and bring hope and healing. In the next chapter, I will describe my research design and methodology on Indo-Guyanese suicides for the period 2010 to 2016.

REFERENCE LIST

Aquinas, T. (n.d.). *Summa Theologica*, Part II-II (Secunda Secundae). Retrieved from http://www.freecatholicebooks.com/books/summa2pt2.pdf

Barraclough, B. (1992). The Bible suicides. *Acta Psychiatrica Scandinavica,* 86(1), 64-69.

Bakke Graduate University. (2017). Transformational leadership perspectives taught at BGU. Retrieved from https://www.bgu.edu/about/eight-transformational-leadership-perspectives-taught-bgu/

Barbour, J. D. (1994). Suicide, tragedy, and theology in "Sophie's Choice" and Gustafson's theocentric ethics. *Literature and Theology*, 8(1), 80–93.

Brown, R. (1999). *Surviving the Loss of a Loved One: living through grief.* Pittsburgh: Autumn House.

Cook, C. C. (2014). Suicide and religion. *The British Journal of Psychiatry*, 204(4), 254–255.

Durkheim, E. (1951). *Suicide: A study in sociology* (JA Spaulding & G. Simpson, trans.). Glencoe, IL: Free Press. *(Original work published 1897)*.

Gavin, D. (2004). From Despair to Hope: A Christian Perspective on the Tragedy of Suicide. Council on Social Responsibility of the Methodist Church in Ireland. *The Furrow,* 55(11), 648–650.

Gearing, R. E. and Lizardi, D. (2009). Religion and suicide. *Journal of Religion and Health*, 48(3), 332-341.

Gill, R. (2006). *A Textbook of Christian ethics.* London: Bloomsbury Publishing.

Gustafson, J. M. 19884. *Ethics from a Theocentric Perspective. Vol. 1, Theology and Ethics. Vol. 2, Ethics and Theology.* Chicago: University of Chicago Press.

Hashmi, A. M., Butt, Z. and Umair, M. (2013). Is depression an inflammatory condition? A review of available evidence. *J Pak Med Assoc*, 63(7), 899-906.

Honderich, T. (ed.) (2005). *The Oxford Companion to Philosophy*. England: Oxford University Press.

Jacobs, L. (1995). *The Jewish Religion: A Companion*. England: Oxford University Press.

Koch, H. J. (2005). Suicides and suicide ideation in the Bible: an empirical survey. *Acta Psychiatrica Scandinavica*, 112(3), 167-172.

Leclaire, J. (2013). Why are so many Pastors committing Suicide? *Charisma News*. https://www.charismanews.com/opinion/watchman-on-the-wall/42063-why-are-so-many-pastors-committing-suicide

Libreria Editrice Vaticana (2003). Cathecism of the Catholic Church. Retrieved from http://www.vatican.va/archive/ENG0015/_INDEX.HTM

London, H. B., & Wiseman, N. B. (2003). *Pastors at greater risk*. CA: Gospel Light Publications.

MacArthur, J. F. (2010). *Called to Lead: 26 Leadership Lessons from the Life of the Apostle Paul*. TN: Thomas Nelson.

McKenzie, N., Baker, R., & Lee, J. (2012). Church's suicide victims. *Canberra Times*. Retrieved from http://www.theage.com.au/frontpage/2012/04/13/frontpage.pdf

Morgan, K. W. (Ed.). (1987). *The Religion of the Hindus*. Delhi: Motilal Banarsidass Publishers.

Mowat, H., Swinton, J., Stark, C., & Mowat, D. (2013). Religion and suicide: Exploring the role of the church in deaths by suicide in Highland, Scotland. *Health Social Care Chaplaincy*, 9(1), 3–7.

Phipps, W. E. (1985). Religion Online. Retrieved from https://www.religion-online.org/article/christian-perspectives-on-suicide/

Pollock, J. (2012). *The Apostle: The Life of Paul*. CO: David C Cook Publishing.

Radhakrishnan, R., & Andrade, C. (2012). Suicide: an Indian perspective. *Indian Journal of Psychiatry*, 54(4), 304–319.

Stack, S. (1983). The effect of religious commitment on suicide: A cross-national analysis. *Journal of Health and Social Behavior*, 24(4), 362–374.

Stack, S. and Wasserman, I. (1992). The effect of religion on suicide ideology: An analysis of the networks perspective. *Journal for the Scientific Study of Religion*, 31(4), 457–466.

World Health Organization. (n.d.). Depression: let's talk. Retrieved from http://www.who.int/topics/depression/en/

PART 4
SUICIDALITY RESEARCH
AND OUTCOMES

CHAPTER 6
PROJECT DESIGN AND RESEARCH METHODOLOGY

"Research is formalized curiosity.
It is poking and prying with a purpose"
(Zora Neale Hurston)

Introduction

This chapter describes the project design and research methodology that were done through an inductive, qualitative research process with Indo-Guyanese suicide attempters and family-member survivors in the five regions in Guyana with the highest suicidality for the period 2010 to 2016. The study focused on (1) collecting data on the pre-and post-suicide attempt life experiences of five suicide attempters, and (2) the stories from family-member survivors relating to the death of five suicide completers. The method of inquiry was a phenomenological reflection and theoretical analysis of the participants' experiences. This method was implemented through an inductive, qualitative research approach, which gives a voice to the participants, while it makes meaning of what is being said from their experiential and psychological perspective. Grounded theory was used to thematically analyze and evaluate the interview data. A consultative process was used to initiate the development of interventions and postventions.

Data Collection

Interview Instrument and Post-Research Evaluation Questionnaire
Firstly, a dual-purpose interview instrument was designed to guide the interview process and capture of interview data from both suicide attempters and family-member survivors. The instrument was used only as a guideline

because the preference was, firstly, to allow participants to share freely about their experiences of the suicide or suicide attempt, and, secondly, to reduce researcher bias. The instrument was structured to capture pre-event, actual day of the event, and post-event life experiences of the participants to get an understanding of the life of the deceased, suicide attempters, and family-member survivors. The instrument was formatted to attract, as far as possible, personal, familial, community, religious and cultural data. It was necessary to edit the instrument after both the first and second interviews because the intermediate analyses showed that other vital information was needed to build on some of the themes that were emerging.

Secondly, a post-research evaluation questionnaire was given to the attendees, during the small group session of the consultation meeting. The aim of the questionnaire was to capture consultation forum members' feedback on the data collection and analysis processes, the research findings, the consultation process, and the need for diffusion of the research findings.

Sample size

Purposive sampling was done, with the sample population taken from within five regions with high completed suicide rates during the period 2010 to 2016. A sample size of ten Indo-Guyanese was chosen for participants to share their stories, five suicide attempters and five family-member survivors. It is not unusual to have such a small sample size for qualitative research, where it is expected each participant to provide and reflect on a detailed account of their lived experience on suicide. The participants were selected because "they 'represent' a perspective, rather than a population" (Smith, et al. 2009, p. 49). Overall, the research was more concerned about, firstly, making meaning of participants' stories by asking intuitive interview questions that penetrated their social lives, and, secondly, highlighting areas that might be deserving of considerable future research. As the study progressed, significant themes started to repeat themselves in the analysis, even cross-regionally, indicating that saturation may have occurred.

Participants

The Guyana Police Force Statistics Department provided me with the suicide data to cover the research period 2010 to 2016. Searches on the internet and some extremely helpful NGOs provided me with useful information that led me to access participants in Regions 2, 3, 4, 5 and 6. All participants were happy to be interviewed and share their experiences. Some participants even commented that the research was very important and necessary.

Interviews

The qualitative research focused on providing understanding and making meaning of the Indo-Guyanese suicide phenomenon by studying the experience of five suicide attempters and five family-member survivors. The actual sites selected for the interviews were based on what was comfortable for the participants. Confidentiality and participant comfort were in situ for all interviews. Qualitative data was gathered face-to-face, audio, and Skype interviews. The interview format was informal, offering confidentiality and a non-judgmental environment to participants. Some empathy and time-out options were interjected during the interviews, as necessary, to help ease participants' pain as they recalled traumatic events. Each taped interview lasted approximately 40 minutes to an hour and was later transcribed verbatim.

Participants were informed of the interview process and were agreeable with the options, specifically that the contents of the interviews will be confidential and that their names would not be disclosed to any third party during the research. Participants were asked if they wanted to be a part of the consultation process when the findings were being presented to relevant professionals who would be instrumental in creating transformational interventions to help to mitigate suicides and ease the grieving process of survivors. The anonymity was extended to participants who wanted to attend the consultation meeting. Offering participants this protective factor was a barrier to the shame and stigma associated with suicide in Guyana and empowered the participants to share freely. Participants were told that the data collected would form a general repository of information on the suicide phenomenon in Guyana, which would help to create effective interventions to mitigate the occurrences of suicides.

Throughout the interviewing process, I endeavoured to keep the discourse open and guided by the participants, asking intuitive questions based on what the participants said, in order to drill down into the participants' lived experiences, and using the interview instrument only as an interview guide. I would then use the data captured in earlier interviews to ask more in-depth open questions if an issue was brought up in subsequent interviews, careful to let the data emerge freely.

I, additionally, interviewed relevant researchers and various NGO staff as well as published authors, all of whom are knowledgeable on the Indo-Guyanese suicide phenomenon. The contributions from the persons interviewed helped in the analysis and understanding of Indo-Guyanese historical, sociological, economical, cultural, and familial issues.

Analysis

Transcripts for the suicide attempters were analyzed to gather information on the perspective of the suicide attempter, whereas family-member survivors' interviews were analyzed to assess the experience of the family-member survivors and provide a psychological autopsy of the suicide victim. All the interview transcripts were meticulously analyzed to systematically produce categories and themes in the development of grounded theory. Noble and Mitchell (2016) describe grounded theory as a research method "concerned with the generation of theory, which is 'grounded' in data that has been systematically collected and analyzed. It is used to uncover such things as social relationships and behaviours of groups, known as social processes" (p. 1).

> Grounded theory is a research method concerned with the generation of theory, which is 'grounded' in data that has been systematically collected and analyzed.

The methodology was mainly developed using Kathy Charmaz's (1990) constructionist version of grounded theory, with some necessary field adjustments I made. I developed a system of listing the different categories that were captured from the interviews and later arranging them into themes to develop a suicide theorization process. Meaning was co-constructed as I worked with two independent individuals to explore cultural context, religiosity, and familial and social complexities that affected how the participants made meaning in their personal lived experiences. Quotations from participants have been included in the findings.

In creating theory, it was important to know whether it was relevant for use in the real world, clear and understandable, and the process could be repeated by another researcher and produce the same findings. It was important not to focus just on data that fitted emerging theory but to be sensitive to all the interview data. As a result, validity was added to the research process.

Added Validity and Rigour

As mentioned earlier, in addition to my personal analysis of the interview data, interview transcripts were also analyzed independently by two individuals, both Guyanese, who not only had cultural connections but who analyzed the transcripts through academic lens. One of the individuals is a Christian pastor, who was previously the Communications Adviser to a former Guyanese President, and the other is a senior official of Guyana's Hindu Dharmic Sabha. The independent feedback from the interview transcripts were recorded and included in the overall schema of making meaning of the suicide phenomenon. The process provided an additional validation layer and rigour (the standards of rigour being credibility, auditability and fittingness, according to Chiovitti and Piran, 2003, p. 434), by buffering the meaning made by participants and reducing researcher bias in the interpretation of the data. Following the steps of the research design and methodology makes it possible for another researcher to repeat my methodology and validate findings through replication.

Intervention Strategy

The consultation process was the method used to determine the intervention strategies needed to help mitigate Indo-Guyanese suicide and support the grieving family-member survivors. Invitations to the consultation meeting were sent to 15 persons who, I believe, could effectively discuss the research findings and contribute towards defining the strategic direction and interventions to mitigate Indo-Guyanese suicides. Eleven persons attended the meeting, and I met with one key decision-maker a day before the meeting for what turned out to be a dry run of the presentation. The meeting was structured in three parts: an initial plenary setting where the problem statement, the research purpose, methodology, and findings were presented, followed by a small group break-out session, structured as two groups of four persons and a group of three persons. Group members discussed and wrote probable intervention strategies in light of the research findings. At the end of the small group discussions, from each small group, a member was chosen to feed back to the larger group the interventions which were discussed. The persons selected for the Consultation meeting, which included doctors, social workers, teachers and counsellors, were capable of introducing some of the interventions (Table 4) discussed into their own sphere of influence. Interventions are planned to be implemented at individual, local/community, regional and national levels.

Table 4

Interventions Suggested by Key Decision-makers at Consultation Meeting

Interventions	Benefits
Men's Forums	To provide guidance and opportunities to share
Counsellors Skilled in General and Grief Counselling	(**For teens**) To provide meaningful friendships based on care, empathy (**For Survivors**) getting intensive help from others
Community Care Groups	Church, parachurch and other organizations
Immediate Care for Victims and Families	To ease the pain and suffering and provide a support mechanism
Coping Strategies	To provide specific support to children but extended to adults
Educating The General Populace About Issues Surrounding Suicides	Knowledge sharing at all levels will provide better understanding of the issues surrounding suicide.
Parenting Skills/Values	To be provided especially to families where children are threatened or at risk from suicide

Reporting All Cases Of Suicide Ideation Or Suicide Attempts	Need to determine the general warning signs for those at risk to suicide and have an accurate system of reporting suicide attempts
Developing A Network And Referrals System	To increase knowledge sharing and provide adequate and relevant support to those exposed to suicide
School-based programs	To provide information and training related to substance abuse, sexuality, help or support systems available at the community level and coping skills
Community-based programs	Training for parents, teachers, health care professionals, police officers on subjects such as mental health, healthy communication, self-esteem and avoidance of stigma, Trades to women in particular.
Improving the Legal Framework	To provide better laws and management of the use of legal and illegal substances
Establish Drug Courts	To manage dispensing of drugs responsibly
Media Reporting	To provide training on responsible media reporting

The consultation meeting provided some key interventions which included men's discussion forums. The forums were intended to provide a platform for men to share the day-to-day challenges they face, given that more men were committing suicide than women. The research found that pesticides were used as a method of committing suicide. Controlled monitoring of the dispensing, use and management of drugs and pesticides is essential and can be attained through improving legislation and working with farmers, pharmacies, and relevant agencies to ensure safety mechanisms are in place. Parenting and coping skills training programs are needed to build and empower stronger families and individuals. Counselling must be done by professionals and include grief counselling for survivors in a preferably group environment.

Additionally, suggestions were made to diffuse the interventions to other agencies, including those who were invited but could not attend the meeting. The diffusion process was not only intended to be within Guyana but to be international so that other researchers and countries could utilize and also build on the research findings.

At an appropriate point of the consultation meeting, the group was tasked with completing a post-research evaluation questionnaire.

Evaluation Methods

The data collection and analysis processes were critical to the production of relevant, integrous, accurate, and unbiased findings. Having a third party process the data and make meaning of what the participants said, independently of the researcher's interpretations, helps to increase validity of the methodology as well as reduce researcher bias.

Additionally, at the consultation meeting, attendees were given a post research evaluation questionnaire to complete, after completion requirements were explained to them. The questionnaire assessed four areas: (1) the overall effectiveness of the research methodology, that is, the effectiveness of the data collection and data analysis processes; (2) the value of the research findings; (3) the effectiveness of the consultation meeting in eliciting interventions; and (4) the need for diffusion of the research finding. The questionnaire used a rating system ranging from a scale of Very Poor to Very Good.

Summary

In this chapter, I have identified the sample of research participants, the data needed for the research, the reason the data was required, and the data collection process. The method of inquiry and analysis were described. I discussed the consultation meeting where the research findings were diffused to the attendees. Some of the practical transformational interventions, and postventions to help mitigate Indo-Guyanese suicides were described. I also described the post-research evaluation questionnaire, which was used to gain feedback on how well the study accomplished its objective. In Chapter 7, I will discuss the outcomes and results of the research described in this chapter.

REFERENCE LIST

Charmaz, K. (1990). 'Discovering' chronic illness: Using grounded theory. *Social Science and Medicine*, 30(11), 1161–1172.

Chiovitti, R. F. and Piran, N. (2003). Rigour and grounded theory research. *Journal of Advanced Nursing*, 44(4), 427–435.

Noble, H. and Mitchell, G. (2016). What is grounded theory?. *Evidence-based nursing*, 19(2), 34-35.

Smith JA, Flowers P. and Larkin M. (2009). *Interpretative phenomenological analysis: Theory, method and research.*

CHAPTER 7
OUTCOMES AND RESULTS

"When people kill themselves, they think they're ending the pain,
but all they're doing is passing it on to those they leave behind."
(Jeannette Walls)

Introduction

This chapter details the outcomes and results of the data collected during
the interviewing of Indo-Guyanese suicide attempters and family-member
survivors. The chapter also discusses the feedback from the consultation
meeting, which was held to diffuse the research findings and initiate intervention strategies to mitigate Indo-Guyanese suicides. In keeping with Kathy
Charmaz's (1990) recommendation for the development of constructivist
grounded theory, I have incorporated some quotes from participants' stories
throughout the chapter to preserve the context and full meaning of the data.
I have also included some feedback from the two independent analyzers of
interview data.

Psychache

Underlying every suicide and suicide attempt is an experience of hopelessness. Generally, hopelessness, disempowerment, misunderstandings and
ruminating thoughts were the basis of the psychache experienced by Indo-
Guyanese suicide attempters and by suicide victims based on a psychological
autopsy with family-member survivors. The two independent analyzers and
I recognized the ongoing mental, emotional, and psychological pain felt by
participants. One independent analyzer, Pastor Oginga reported:

What I have been able to gather from these interviews is that they more or less present an aggregate... of the pains that lead up to suicide. What I am gathering from participants is that these pains remain long after the act is committed in the minds of those who have been affected.

The pain felt was expressed through words such as loneliness, brokenness, depression, and self-hate. When discussing her experiences that included sexual abuse from family members and led her to frequent suicide attempts, one participant stated,

Because of my past, I normally get breakdowns, which means I cry myself to sleep. I get depressed. I attempted suicide a lot. I used to cut... I normally tell my friends physically, I am really, really strong, but mentally, I'm like an eggshell, a broken one.

On reflecting on the suicide of her boyfriend, one participant stated, "Time does not heal... Every day is worse." One family-member survivor displayed deep pain of suddenly losing a loved one when she shared, "I didn't want to live anymore... I couldn't bear it anymore. It was so hard."

Pain was clearly evident with all but one participant as participants mostly cried throughout the interviews. The participant who did not weep had firmly resolved to put her brother's suicide behind her and move forward. Her brother had committed suicide, at age 17, and her mother blamed her father for speaking harshly to her brother to get him to leave the 'rum shop' where he was imbibing alcohol with his friends as he mourned the death of a close family member. The frequent arguments between her parents over her brother's suicide had ended in separation, and she was left at home to take care of her father.

Overall, suicide attempters and family-member survivors have experienced great pain, a situation which was confirmed by one of the independent analyzers. According to Pompili, Lester, Leenaars, Tatarelli and Girardi (2008), the wisdom of suicidology shows that suicide individuals are experiencing great psychological pain and that suicide may, in part, be an attempt to escape from the unendurable suffering (p. 116).

Two instruments guided the development of the interview instrument used in the research. The first instrument was Shneidman's (1999) Psychological

Pain Assessment Scale, which was developed to measure the psychache and potentially identify persons at risk for suicide (p. 287). The second instrument was Beck, Weissman, Lester, and Trexler's (1974) Beck Hopelessness Scale (BHS), a 20-item true or false questionnaire designed to measures aspects of hopelessness or pessimism. The BHS records feelings about the future, loss of motivation and expectations to present a picture of the level of hopelessness being experienced by the individual (pp. 861–862). The research found that psychache and hopelessness highly correlate with suicide intent as discussed earlier.

Types of Suicide Identified

Two types of suicides have been revealed from participants' stories: the planned suicide and the spontaneous suicide. In planned suicides, the person tended to signal intent by getting rid of possessions, bringing an end to personal long-term or routine operations, focusing on timeframes given that the demise date is decided, telling others of the suicide plan and/or leaving a suicide note or message. In addition, the individual's behaviour or mood tended to change abruptly closer to the suicide date/time, often to a more cheerful or thoughtful disposition. The research found that although suicide victims who plan their suicides want to die, they also want others to have good memories of them after their demise.

In spontaneous suicides, the person, often a young person, often acts on a momentary impulsive decision. Impulsive suicide attempters were influenced by alcohol and drug abuse, childhood sexual abuse, harsh words, turbulent or angry household, and misunderstandings between parents and children. In addition to types of suicides, the methods used to commit suicide were evident.

Methods Used to Commit Suicide

The research found that although hanging was used by one male suicide completer, most suicide attempters and completers ingested poison, such as Gramoxone, Agra Zone and Bestac, which are agrochemicals intended for use on farmlands. Many Indo-Guyanese in the research regions are farmers and store the poisonous agrochemicals in refrigerators, which are often easily accessible. After ingesting poison, one participant claimed that she had "No regrets for attempting suicide except for having to deal with the pain of the poison."

According to one of the independent analyzers, there was a government campaign initiated by former Minister of Health, and a community programme also involving the Ministry of Health, to secure the poisonous substances in a white cupboard with double locks. However, the initiatives are no longer functioning effectively.

> Over the period 2010 to 2015, more males attempted suicides than females. However, in 2014 and 2015, the female/male suicide ratio continued to increase until in 2016, more females attempted suicides than males.

Other methods of attempted suicide included ingesting large quantities of paracetamol and valium, prescriptive drugs which in one case had been dispensed directly by a pharmacy to a minor. From this example, it is clear that pharmacy regulations and controls are either not in place or not being adhered to. Pharmacists in Guyana are meant to follow the Pharmacy Practitioners Act of Guyana 2003. I spoke with one pharmacist about the dispensing of prescribed drugs to minors, and although there was recognition that the Pharmacy Practitioners Act of Guyana 2003 dictates that a minor must always be accompanied by an adult, there is no national guarantee that all pharmacists adopt the policy.

Male/Female Suicide Ratio

From the research data provided by the Guyana Police Force for the period 2010 to 2016, more men have consistently *committed* suicides than women (Figure 9), and they were more intentional about ending their lives, choosing methods such as hanging and fatal poisons. My attempts throughout the research to interview more men proved futile. Family-member survivors of suicide victims readily came forward, but in two cases of young men age 17 who committed suicide, one having died over ten years ago and the other three years ago, both survivors shared that they wanted to forget the incidents. The remaining suicides occurred within the last three months.

Over the period 2010 to 2015, more males *attempted* suicides than females.

However, in 2014 and 2015, the female/male suicide ratio continued to increase until in 2016, more females attempted suicides than males. Additionally, 2016 saw more female suicides than the two previous years. The statistics show that in 2016, more females committed and attempted suicide. Between 2014 and 2016, male suicides decreased very slightly, male suicide attempts remained roughly around the same level. Overall, although male Indo-Guyanese suicides have been decreasing, on average, the number of Indo-Guyanese female suicides has remained about the same.

2016 saw more female suicides than the two previous years. The statistics show that in 2016, more females committed and attempted suicide. Between 2014 and 2016, male suicides decreased very slightly, male suicide attempts remained roughly around the same level.

The females who came forward to be interviewed were aged between 16 and 51, with most attempters, ages below 20 years. Family-member survivors were also mostly females who spoke of the deaths of male relatives.

Reasons Proffered for Suicide Attempts and Actual Suicides

Overwhelming emotions; abuse, which include substance abuse; depression; misunderstanding, and family dysfunction.

A number of reasons were revealed for suicide attempts and actual suicides during the interviews. The reasons included overwhelming emotions; abuse, which include substance abuse; depression; misunderstanding, and family dysfunction.

Overwhelming Emotions

Spontaneous suicides were triggered by momentary, overwhelming emotions such as anger, frustration, and/or fear, usually a result of experiencing harsh words. One participant committed suicide because of the anger and frustration he felt when harsh words were spoken to him by a parent. Being the target of the irresponsible use of social media also led to suicide. Social media has been used to adversely affect a participant's self-image, and generate fear and confusion. Additionally, constant quarrelling or abusive behaviours within the family have created household turbulence and led to suicide and suicide attempts.

Some spontaneous suicide attempters said they really did not want to die. One attempter admitted it was a mistake to attempt suicide but was overwhelmed by situational emotions.

> Some spontaneous suicide attempters said they really did not want to die.

Participants from planned and spontaneous suicides felt hopeless and/or disempowered. One suicide attempter experienced overwhelming helplessness as she watched her angry father beat her disabled brother. To bring an end to the assault the participant picked up a knife and cried, "Dad if you [continue to] beat this boy I will kill myself."

Abuse (including substance abuse)

According to family-member survivors interviewed, experiences of the suicide victims included domestic violence; peer abuse, which destroyed the victim's self-image and self-confidence, family conflicts, estrangement from loved ones for reasons such as a lack of understanding of the victim's perspective; emotional isolation; physical separation from young children, and feelings of rejection and exclusion in that victims felt they were no longer needed by their families. Some spontaneous suicide victims were under the influence of excessive alcohol. One suicide victim was being physically and emotionally abused by her boyfriend, who was abusing drugs.

Depression and Misunderstanding

One participant, who has attempted suicide three times, being unable to deal with the death by suicide of her boyfriend, stated, "It's too much to bear. It's too much to cry out. I didn't feel comfortable being alone... nobody understood. They said 'Stop crying. You can't live this way,' but they never tried to understand how I feel."

> It's too much to bear. It's too much to cry out. I didn't feel comfortable being alone... nobody understood. They said 'Stop crying. You can't live this way,' but they never tried to understand how I feel.

Family dysfunction

This study found that family conflicts constituted most of the suicides or suicide attempts. Family conflicts included disagreements with key family members because of perceived harsh words used for reprimanding the participant or suicide victim. There were also unhealthy relationships between parents and children and unhealthy relational dependence between partners. Cultural clashes were found between children and parents. There was spousal abuse, and incest was discovered in one case. Mothers were often absent from the homes because they were working long hours away from home or had migrated overseas. All participants had experienced multiple adverse life incidences; for example, one young participant life span experiences included sexual abuse, self-harming, ingesting alcohol from the age of 12, and domestic child abuse. The research findings align with the study from Dube et al. (2001) that found

> adverse childhood experiences dramatically increase the risk of attempting suicide....recognition that adverse childhood experiences are common and frequently take place as multiple events may be the first step in preventing their occurrence; identifying and treating persons who have been affected by such experiences may have substantial value in our evolving efforts to prevent suicide. (p. 7)

I explored the relationship between anger, frustration, and pain to see how this was aligned to my thought that the pain of psychache drives suicide. From my counselling experience, I am aware that frustration gradually builds up to anger if left unchecked, and stems mostly from unmet needs. Anger and pain are closely linked because pain affects the emotions. Emotions play a significant role in the pain experience in that psychic pain fuels anger, which in turn may cause, for example, depression, particularly if repressed;

and social detachment or active retaliation against self or others. Therefore frustration, anger, and pain are interrelated and is a potential for suicide. A study by Fernandez (2005) states that:

> anger is a subjective feeling of unpleasantness originating from attributions of wrongdoing and accompanied by tendencies toward retaliation... The subjective feeling of anger ranges in intensity from annoyance or irritation to fury or rage. This intensity is correlated with autonomic arousal... its display is a form of social communication. This functionalist perspective helps us make sense of the anger of those in pain... Anger usually is directed at the one committing the wrongdoing and, in the context of pain, that target is the person responsible for the injury or disease. Theoretically, this can be the self, but there is a common proclivity to blame others for one's pain...or other suffering and setbacks. (p. 101)

There was evident family dysfunction where husbands who were the sole breadwinners did not support their wives financially, and as a result, the wives had to seek employment, which for some meant long periods away from home. Some husbands were challenged by the abuse of alcohol, not helped by the ease of access to the substance. Some minors drank alcohol while still attending school. The use of drugs such as marijuana also contributed to negative behaviour within families which triggered suicide attempts. According to one analyzer:

There's a lack of recreation across board. And many people use alcohol as a sort of cultural escape, culture in the sense of Guyana culture. That is the fittest thing they can do, whether they drink at home socially with friends or go out and do it. It is something that is very accepted and now, to me, it's become something that is totally out of control. Younger and younger people are drinking alcohol because it's a legal substance in a sense. Unlike things like cocaine and marijuana, you can get alcohol legally at any age, except those who are underage. There's no good enforcement of the laws when it comes to alcohol...I'm seeing the social erosion it's causing in society.

> Many people use alcohol as a sort of cultural escape, culture in the sense of Guyana culture.

Indo-Guyanese families are structured around the patriarchal system. Three participants shared that mothers had to seek employment in order to meet their financial needs because the fathers who were the sole breadwinners did not provide for their wives financially. The females were forced to seek employment, working long hours away from the home, all three of the women travelling overseas, with one doing menial work in Surinam in order to sustain the family's income. Often the mothers' departures have left children and young adults in the care of fathers who expect the children to take care of the home. One young participant stated, "I am trying my best to do everything and try to please [everyone] at the same time... it makes me feel as if I'm just there, like they just have me because they got me... who forgets their child's birthday?"

> I am trying my best to do everything and try to please [everyone] at the same time... it makes me feel as if I'm just there, like they just have me because they got me... who forgets their child's birthday?

Young participants in dysfunctional families have reported witnessing physical abuse and constant arguments not only between the parents but between siblings and parents. Often expletives were used by parents in front of their offspring, and on one occasion, a glass object was thrown by a male at his mother.

In describing her experience, one participant reflected on her father's actions: "Ever since I know myself he's been beating and cursing my Mum... constantly cursing. It kind of messes with your brain and at some point, you can't deal with that." When asked the reason for attempting suicide, the same participant stated, "I guess because I just wanted some peace and quiet so I took [the pills]". The participant's home environment was described as turbulent, where the father and one male sibling did most of the screaming at the females. The participant was made to do arduous and some unpleasant domestic chores.

> Some young adults believed they were misunderstood and not loved by their parents.

Additionally, the research found that young people were not talking to their parents about their problems because they claim when they do share what is happening, they felt misunderstood or not taken seriously. Communication within the dysfunctional families often deteriorated to the point where family members did not know what other family members were dealing with. Some young adults believed they were misunderstood and not loved by their parents. One participant who frequently attempted suicide, medicated on alcohol as a minor to ease the pain of being sexually abused as a child. In discussing the abuse, the participant stated:

> When I told my Mum… what happened to me, she would start arguing saying she doesn't know why I'm behaving like that. I would tell her that 'You know exactly why I'm behaving like that'. She would say 'What do you want me to do? I can't do anything about it. I don't care'… That hurt a lot… it hurts so much. They never said they wanted me to be like [my sister] but that's the way I feel. She's the perfect child. She doesn't say anything. She goes into her room and cuts her hand. Interviewer: 'She does what?' Participant: She cuts her wrist.

Stigma

Some participants stated they experienced various degrees of stigma, such as stigma of being in hospital knowing that the circumstance of their admission engendered guilt and shame. In order to avoid the shame felt over her child's suicide attempt, one mother 'self-discharged' her minor, although the child needed necessary hospital care. There were no indications that the community shuns those who attempted suicide. Instead, the interview found that the church, where Christian Indo-Guyanese committed suicide, and community members, showed concern and compassion towards grieving family-member survivors.

Stigma of being in hospital knowing that the circumstance of their admission engendered guilt and shame.

One participant, a 20-year old male, claimed that he had no intention of committing suicide when he drank from a bottle of kerosene, which he claimed he mistook for water. Kerosene has a very pungent smell. On investigation, I was informed by the medical profession that it was normal for a suicide attempter to make such a claim because of the stigma attached to suicide and because suicide is still considered a criminal offence.

One family-member survivor mentioned that her daughter who committed suicide was told by hospital staff that on leaving hospital she would be

> The stigma of suicide and the criminal charge associated with suicide are huge barriers to healing of psychache.

sent to prison for the crime. As a result, the suicide completer refused her medication and died soon after.

The stigma of suicide and the criminal charge associated with suicide are huge barriers to healing of psychache and are therefore issues which require urgent attention. The criminal charge has not proved to be an effective deterrent in reducing suicides and is, in fact, preventing those who really need help from seeking support.

Grieving Process

In all cases, the interviews revealed that where there was a death due to suicide, the grieving process left family-member survivors not only distressed but with many unanswered questions. Survivors who had recently experience loss were at the initial stage of the grieving cycle, with many overwhelmed or confused over the death. Survivors could not understand why their loved ones had chosen to end their lives by suicide; they experienced guilt and

> Where there was a death due to suicide, the grieving process left family-member survivors not only distressed but with many unanswered questions.

blamed themselves for not being able to do something to stop the suicide. Survivors believed that if they knew the suicide was about to occur they would have intervened to stop it and blamed themselves because they could not stop the suicide. However, some victims did indicate their intention to kill themselves to survivors at a time prior to the actual suicide, and on hindsight, survivors said there were some clear signs as to the intention of suicide, but they did not take them seriously.

> Survivors believed that if they knew the suicide was about to occur they would have intervened to stop it and blamed themselves because they could not stop the suicide.

The grieving stage was different for each participant who experienced a loss. A family-member survivor, who experienced the death of a brother, and a suicide attempter, who experienced the loss of a loved one at approximately the same timeframe, were both at different stages of the grieving cycle. The family-member survivor in question was trying to move forward by putting the episode behind her while the attempter was having ruminating thoughts, experiencing the pain of the memories that caused her to have multiple attempts at suicide. One participant stated, "The more the days go by the more you're thinking about it... it's just something that eats you, it just sucks you."

According to Jordan (2009), death by suicide can be mysterious, leaving survivors to make meaning of what has taken place, why it has occurred, who is 'responsible' for the death, and their perceived relationship with the deceased. Survivors perform their personal psychological autopsy "into the state of mind of the deceased and the factors that led to the suicide. This includes an accounting of the survivor's own perceived responsibility for the death and their perceived failure to prevent the suicide" (p. 6).

Sands (2009) states:

> As the bereaved begin to reconstruct the death story they find themselves *walking in the shoes* of the deceased, trying to make meaning of the pain in the deceased's life and death. These meaning making activities are relational and challenge the relationship with the self, the deceased and significant others. Analysis identified the prevalence of the bereaved forming maladaptive relationships with the deceased. The intense focus and rumination on reconstruction can increase the vulnerability of the bereaved to suicidal ideation and possible suicide. (p. 15)

It is, therefore, important for health care providers to know that survivors may be prone to suicide, and survivors must be helped to realistically balance their perspectives as they work to make meaning of their loss. Therefore, effect support systems must be in place.

Support Systems

All the young suicide attempters expressed the pain of being misunderstood and unsupported by parents. Some participants felt there was no place they could go to feel supported in difficult times, which made them feel even more isolated. One participant stated that after attempting suicide, she was lonely in the hospital because of restriction on her visitors. Another participant found comfort in being helped by an NGO to find activities that provided distractions, and she was able to say, "I'm engaging myself in other things, what I like." The NGO has helped to prevent her from spending time alone doing only routine things, a situation which for some previous suicide attempters poses an additional risk for re-attempt. Change and activities which create distractions have helped attempters to think about different things.

The study found that none of the participants received formal counselling sessions apart from those who spoke with social workers while in hospital. One social worker informed me that one of his roles was to engage where necessary with Child Protection and other agencies before allowing re-entry into the attempter's usual environment. Some family-member survivors did not know that such help was available, and like other participants, they also wanted to have counselling support publicized and made available.

One risk factor for suicide attempters who have not received effective support stems from their returning back into the same environment in which they experienced abuse. Being unable to discuss the cause for the attempt can make them isolated and therefore vulnerable to other suicide attempts.

Socialization

Some participants described themselves as 'loners' who rarely socialized or discussed their experiences in their homes with an external party or peers. One of the independent analyzers for the interview transcripts noted that in one location, the routine for many individuals in the community was home, to school or work, then return to home. There were no recreational facilities in the area, and it was not unusual for alcohol to be imbibed in the home on a regular basis. One 16-year-old participant claimed that she was not allowed to have male friends, and when the only female friend she had visited, she would go into her room because her friend was afraid of her father.

A young Christian participant who attempted suicide has been living with her grandparents, who are Hindus, from an early age after her parents separated. The minor stated she stayed in her room most of the time to avoid the frequent arguments with her grandparents relating to her school. The young lady participated in minimal Hindu ceremonial activities with her grandparents but said she was experiencing a lot of anger for having to live under the conditions. One suicide attempter, who stated she did not socialize, not only showed evidence of self-harming when difficulties arose in the home, the indicated that her sibling, who also did not socialize, was also self-harming when there was family conflict. Three suicide attempters stated that they did not socialize much but would mostly stay in their rooms when at home. Generally, there is a lack of recreation facilities across the five regions, which has affected community socialization, with more and more persons becoming socially isolated.

> Generally, there is a lack of recreation facilities across the five regions, which has affected community socialization, with more and more persons becoming socially isolated.

Suicide Messages

In only one case was a suicide message left, and the message was left in the form of a song. One young Christian repeat attempter said she always prayed for forgiveness from those she ever hurt and forgave all whoever hurt her prior to ingesting large quantities of drugs that should not have been prescribed to a minor.

Religion

Not all of the Indo-Guyanese participants were Hindus; some were Christians. One Christian Indo-Guyanese suicide completer's mother was left questioning why she would commit such an act and blames it on her association with a 'new' Hindu boyfriend who was not only a drug abuser and physically abused her daughter but who, according to the distraught mother, on the day of the incident, watched her pour out the poison and walked away as she drank it. The survivor

> Not all of the Indo-Guyanese participants were Hindus; some were Christians.

mother was also exposed to domestic violence from her husband whom she claimed drank '24/7' and was also unemployed.

Both Hindus and Christians are taught as part of their religious belief system about the value of life, that life is a precious gift. From my study, however, I observed how the meaning of life is devalued when it comes up against coping with psychache. In their own strengths, the victims' pain threshold cannot withstand the pain associated with hopelessness. Essentially, the lack of coping skills drove young people as well as adults to commit or attempt suicide. This situation raises genuine questions in terms of the depth of some Christians' understanding of the hope which is promised in the Bible when faced with trials and also on reflection of Apostle Paul's examples of his trials.

Police and Health Care Providers

As mentioned earlier, one mother claimed her daughter gave up the fight to live because her daughter was told by hospital staff she would be imprisoned for six years when she got better. One family-member survivor said that police, who attended the scene of a relative's hanging, did not want to remove the deceased as he hung from a tree but asked a family-member to do so and also asked to use the family member's telephone to make a call to the morgue because the police did not have credits to make the call. First responders and care givers have an important duty towards those under their care and should be fully cognizant of how to provide an efficient and effective service at all times.

First responders and care givers have an important duty towards those under their care and should be fully cognizant of how to provide an efficient and effective service at all times.

Risk factors

The research highlighted certain risk factors which included previous suicide attempts, easy access to poison, and items classified as prescriptive drugs. One person succeeded in completing the suicide act after two attempts, whereas another suicide attempter has so far repeated the act three times within two years. Depression was another risk factor evidenced in a multiple repeat attempter. Stress was also presented as a factor that led to suicide.

> Certain risk factors ... included previous suicide attempts, easy access to poison, and items classified as prescriptive drugs.

One participant, whose attempt at suicide included self-harming by cutting around the veins on her wrists, stated that her sister was also self-harming. One of the independent analyzers, Dr. X, noted that if a family-member has attempted or committed suicide "the risk of attempt by another (*family member*) is high, and not even in the family but people in the community."

> The risk of attempt by another (family member) is high, and not even in the family but people in the community.

Consultative Process

The research findings were shared at a consultation meeting (Table 5), to which 15 key stakeholders were invited, but 11 attended. I also met with one stakeholder separately. The findings were first presented and discussed at both plenary and small group levels, with small groups instructed to develop and feedback interventions to the plenary level. The feedback of interventions is shown in Table 4.

Table 5

Consultation Meeting Agenda

12.00 – 12.30 Registration	
PART 1: 12.30 – 1.00pm	**PART 2: 1.00 – 1.45pm**
1. Introductions	7. Small group discussion of research findings
2. Objective of the Meeting	
3. Overview of the Indo-Guyanese Suicide Phenomenon with History & Statistics	8. Small group discussion of possible Interventions to mitigate suicide based on research findings
4. Objective of the Research	9. Evaluation Questionnaires for completion
5. Research Design & Methodology	**PART 3: 1.45 – 2.30pm**
6. Research Findings	10. Feedback of possible Interventions from Part 2 to plenary setting
OTHER:	
Attendance Sheet	11. Proposed next steps
Light Refreshments	12. Thanks and Close

A number of transformational interventions were suggested by the key stakeholders (Table 4). Interventions included having a platform for men to share what challenges they faced, given that more men were committing suicide. Support systems including advocacy and general and grief counselling must be available for all suicide attempters and family-member survivors, with networking and referral systems incorporated so that relevant agencies may interact. Education and training must be an essential part of the transformational process, extending from the individual to the national level and beyond and must include coping strategies to reorient parents and reintegrate families, to assist teachers, Health Care providers, the police, pharmacies, government and legal arms to ensure the better management of legal and illegal substances. The programs must be school and community based. There must also be very intensive training to ensure the media reports on suicide responsibly.

Meeting members were also asked to complete a project evaluation questionnaire. Overall, meeting members believed that the research and consultation processes achieved the set objectives, and a number of recommendations were made to encourage diffusion of the findings to achieve fuller impact and increase transformation.

Summary

In this chapter, I have identified in depth the results of the data collection process. In summary, suicide is a major public health issue. The research shows that Indo-Guyanese suicides and attempted suicides were a response to the participant's exposure, environment, upbringing, socialization, value systems, psychological makeup, and coping skills. All of these conditions interrelate to create movement towards suicide. The decision made to commit suicide is multifaceted, crossing the boundaries of existing psychosocial theories but having at its foundation, Shneidman's (1993) theory of psychache, a psychological pain that surpasses their coping capability, making them feel they are incapable of resolving their problems.

I have also described the intervention and postvention strategies developed at the consultation meeting which will help to mitigate Indo-Guyanese suicides. I have also highlighted the feedback I received from the Consultation meeting as post-research evaluation. In Chapter 8, I will provide some concluding remarks and describe implications of my research.

REFERENCE LIST

Beck, A. T., Schuyler, D. and Herman, I. (1974). *Development of suicidal intent scales*. England: Charles Press Publishers.

Charmaz, K. (1990). 'Discovering' chronic illness: Using grounded theory. *Social Science and Medicine*, 30(11), 1161–1172.

Dube, S. R., Anda, R. F., Felitti, V. J., Chapman, D. P., Williamson, D. F. and Giles, W. H. (2001). Childhood abuse, household dysfunction, and the risk of attempted suicide throughout the life span: findings from the adverse childhood experiences study. *Jama*, 286(24), 3089–3096.

Fernandez, E. (2005). The relationship between anger and pain. *Current Pain and Headache Reports*, 9(2), 101–105.

Jordan, J. R. (2009). After suicide: Clinical work with survivors. *Grief Matters: The Australian Journal of Grief and Bereavement*, 12(1), 4–9.

Pompili, M., Lester, D., Leenaars, A. A., Tatarelli, R. and Girardi, P. (2008). Psychache and suicide: a preliminary investigation. *Suicide and Life-Threatening Behavior*, 38(1), 116–121.

Sands, D. (2009). A tripartite model of suicide grief: Meaning-making and the relationship with the deceased. *Grief Matters: The Australian Journal of Grief and Bereavement*, 12(1), 10.

Shneidman, E. S. (1993). Commentary: Suicide as psychache. *The Journal of Nervous and Mental disease*, 181(3), 145–147.

Shneidman, E. S. (1999). The psychological pain assessment scale. *Suicide and Life-Threatening Behavior*, 29(4), 287–294.

PART 5
RESEARCH CONCLUSIONS

CHAPTER 8
CONCLUSIONS AND IMPLICATIONS

"I'm like an eggshell, a broken one."
(Research Participant)

Introduction

This chapter concludes the research findings and highlights the implications of these findings. It summarizes the principles learnt from the study and discusses possible areas for future research. I also offer some concluding observations as I reflect on the research.

Research Objective

The phenomenological, qualitative research set out to provide understanding of the lived experiences of Indo-Guyanese suicide attempters and family-member survivors of suicide completers in five of Guyana's regions with the highest suicidality during 2010 and 2016. I believe that the research objective has been attained because it has provided a platform for suicide attempters and family-member survivors to voice their stories through their lived experiences. Additionally, the grounded theory process enabled meaning to be made of the suicide phenomenon and causes and consequences were identified.

Consultation Outcomes

Based on the research findings, strategic transformational interventions were developed to help mitigate suicide and to implement relevant support mechanisms to improve the lives of suicide attempters and grieving family-member survivors. The consultation meeting comprised of multiple-discipline key stakeholders, who are not only intentional about mitigating Indo-Guyanese suicides but want to see the findings diffused to and adopted by all relevant agencies. Additionally, because of the research design and methodology employed, the research findings provide a platform for further inductive research not only on Indo-Guyanese suicides but on the full gamut of suicides in Guyana.

Summary of Principles Learnt

Suicide is a major public health issue. The research shows that Indo-Guyanese suicides and attempted suicides were a response to factors such as the participant's exposure to psychache, hopelessness, their environment, upbringing, socialization, value systems, psychological makeup and coping skills. All of these conditions interrelate to create movement towards suicide. Prinstein (2008) noted,

few theoretical models have been offered to help understand self-injury in the manner that other manifestations of psychopathology have been examined. In particular, few studies have considered integrative models that address interplay between dynamic systems within the individual and between individuals and their environments. (p. 2)

In seeking to develop theory on the Indo-Guyanese suicides, without formally creating a theory, I believe that the phenomenological research has elucidated that the decision made to commit suicide is multifaceted, crossing the boundaries of existing psychosocial theories but having at its foundation, Shneidman's (1993) theory of psychache, a psychological pain that surpasses their coping capability, making them feel they are incapable of resolving their problems.

Psychache creates such an intense mental and soul-ish state of hopelessness, such that suicide attempters feel an escape from life is needed. I believe this state is more than depression that may be medicated to make the sufferer at least feel better for a time. However, this state encompasses unendurable pain, loneliness, brokenness, and as one participant aptly described,

"I'm like an eggshell, a broken one." Interview data showed there are levels of mental, emotional and psychological intensity of the state depending on the challenge faced by the individual, the individual's capacity to cope, and that determines how successful the attempt is. Perhaps it may seem to some that the Indo-Guyanese men who choose hanging may have an additional challenge in setting up a noose prior to the suicide, as opposed to a school child who takes 60 paracetamols impulsively. However, for each person the journey to attempting suicide crosses pain thresholds that are unbearable and beyond personal coping capability.

The study has shown that when participants are faced with psychache, there is no capacity to cope with the challenge being faced, and particularly where there are no effective support systems to reach out to, suicide becomes the participant's pain release of choice. This level of dilemma extends from the school child to the full grown working adult.

Not forgetting the psychache being experienced by Indo-Guyanese Christian suicide attempters and completers, the study does raise the concern about the value placed on life in the presence of suffering. How far away from the pained mind and heart is the understanding of the available assurance of hope and God's protection mentioned for Christian believers in Scriptures such as:

All praise to God, the Father of our Lord Jesus Christ. It is by his great mercy that we have been born again, because God raised Jesus Christ from the dead. Now we live with great expectation, and we have a priceless inheritance—an inheritance that is kept in heaven for you, pure and undefiled, beyond the reach of change and decay. And through your faith, God is protecting you by his power until you receive this salvation, which is ready to be revealed on the last day for all to see. (1 Peter 1:3–5 NLT)

Because of our faith, Christ has brought us into this place of unde-served privilege where we now stand, and we confidently and joyfully look forward to sharing God's glory. We can rejoice, too, when we run into problems and trials, for we know that they help us develop endurance. And endurance develops strength of character, and char-acter strengthens our confident hope of salvation. And this hope will not lead to disappointment. For we know how dearly God loves us, because he has given us the Holy Spirit to fill our hearts with his love. When we were utterly helpless, Christ came at just the right time and died for us sinners. (Romans 5:2–6 NLT)

As a result of the research findings, I wonder what factor must be present for Indo-Guyanese Christians to be truly joyful while they endure many trials. There is a conscious decision by suicide victims to prefer the pain of hanging or ingesting poison or large quantities of prescriptive drugs as opposed to experiencing the pain of their circumstances. In terms of Hindu Indo-Guyanese and the valuing of life, one of the analyzers stated:

> As we advance, technology is redefining life on earth. Similarly when traditions are producing negative effects we must understand there is something that needs correcting... show (people) the alternative can work better than their way...
> I won't tell you not to believe in reincarnation because you will take my head but I can tell you while you are in this carnation you have a value, meaning, purpose which can only come out when you're under pressure, when some kind of challenge comes up. It's in the face of challenge that you know who you really are.

What is clear from the research findings is that there is a lot of pain and suffering associated with suicide and attempted suicide, including the distress felt by family-member survivors, and often extended to the community, sometimes long after the incident has occurred. According to Peltz (2017):

> In the human life-cycle people are born, they reproduce, and pass away in older years. Clearly a multitude of events can take place during a lifespan to disrupt that pattern, which is often the case. However, choosing to end one's life early has become a serious health problem and causes hardships and trauma to surviving family members, as well as to the community. (p. 5)

Choosing to end one's life early has become a serious health problem and causes hardships and trauma to surviving family members, as well as to the community.

My study found that participants have experienced the pain of hopelessness as a result of combinations of abusive relationships; rejection; misunderstandings, often as a result of a disconnect or unaligned perspectives on events; difficult parent-child and parent-parent relationships, leading to household dysfunction; a lack of socialization skills, all of which create a sense of thwarted belongingness.

The Interpersonal Theory of Suicide by Van Orden et al. (2010) states:

We propose that the most dangerous form of suicidal desire is caused by the simultaneous presence of two interpersonal constructs—thwarted belongingness and perceived burdensomeness (and hopelessness about these states)—and further, that the capability to engage in suicidal behavior is separate from the desire to engage in suicidal behavior. According to the theory, the capability for suicidal behavior emerges, via habituation and opponent processes, in response to repeated exposure to physically painful and/or fear-inducing experiences. (p. 1)

Indo-Guyanese individuals and families are suffering from multifaceted personal and familial challenges respectively, and younger and younger persons are being affected. Addressing the fundamental issues are just as important, if not more important, as medicating the mental health challenge. Targeted interventions included counselling, particularly grief counselling, and cognitive behavioural therapy. School and community-based programs were needed to trigger the awareness of the seriousness of suicide on both a community and a national level. Programs were needed to provide parenting and coping skills, and for teachers, health care providers, government and legal professionals, and first level suicide responders to respond effectively and efficiently to all incidents of suicide and suicide attempts. The interventions are all crucial first steps in moving forward to shalom and the mitigation of suicides.

Indo-Guyanese men need to have a special focus such as a platform in men's forums. More males than females are committing suicide, but, as mentioned earlier, I have found that the males are unwilling to come forward under the research lens.

My study has shown a challenge to the Indo-Guyanese family structure that has been mainly patriarchal, with fathers working to provide for the family and mothers more involved with domestic roles within the homes. Now, more women are seeking employment away from the family home for long periods, often working to supplement the family income, especially where men are not contributing as expected to the financial upkeep of the family. This shift has weakened the family structure and as such requires urgent reparative attention, which may mean, for example, women being trained in areas where they can find or create jobs that they can perform nearer to or within the home and also a fairer distribution of work within the home.

Alcohol plays a major predisposing role in Indo-Guyanese suicides, evidenced by school-age children drinking heavily. Sometimes alcohol is either abused by the victim or being abused by someone else who then abuses the victim. Where alcohol has proved to be a problem, the household is turbulent, with abusive and violent behaviours exhibited by parents and witnessed by their children. According to Pompili et al. (2010):

Alcohol abuse is a means of easing one's psychological stress but, at the same time, impacts on all other factors, rendering suicide more likely... Suicidal behavior usually occurs early in the course of mood disorders, but only in the final phase of alcohol abuse when social marginalization and poverty, the somatic complications of alcoholism and the breakdown of important social bonds have taken over. (p. 1414) By implication, the link between suicide and alcohol requires steps to be taken to ensure responsible drinking, such as education programs to raise awareness of the dangers of excessive alcohol usage. Interventions may also include public health laws passed or enforced for legal alcohol limits, age-related purchase of alcohol, clear opening and closing times for facilities that sell alcohol, employers frequently testing the blood alcohol levels of those prone to alcohol, and having a corrective system in place.

The study found that many young people are attempting and committing mostly spontaneous suicide. Indo-Guyanese lives are cut short and so are the many productive years that could have been used to fulfill personal purpose and contribute to the development of the nation. The interviews have shown that the young people attempting and committing suicide have poor socializing skills and tended to spend much time on their own. Socializing skills need to be developed through self-confidence, self-esteem and self-image activities. Schools may be instrumental in creating curricula that develop young people in these areas. In speaking of the potentially positive roles of schools in assisting students to socialize, Barnová and Gabrhelová (2017) state:

> Their attempt is to prepare students which can integrate into other social structures and are able to adapt to new social environments. It is not possible to achieve without teaching children and youth to cope with adversity occurring in their social ecologies. (p. 7)

Recreation facilities need to be made available, generally, across Guyana's regions. Additionally, when young people and adults state they will commit suicide, it must be taken seriously. Family-member survivors are shocked when the threat actualizes and they are left with many unanswered questions.

We don't have enough research in the country to guide policy, legislation, anything... Checks and enforcements are needed for Pharmacy regulations and regulations of the Poison Pesticides Board, especially for controlled substances.

My study, however, has shown that there is a relationship between a person's exposure to abuse and dysfunction within the home to suicide; therefore, if someone who possesses these risk factors threatens suicide, it is a clear signal about suicide ideation that should trigger the involvement of support systems in the form of qualified, experienced health care professionals. Generally, there must be mental health and self-awareness programs with confidentiality as a vital component. Fleischmann et al. (2008) recommend a support system such as "a 'tele-help/ tele-check' service (i.e. an alarm system that can be activated to call for help and a service that contacts a person twice a week for assessment of their needs and to provide emotional support)" (p. 704).

Throughout the interviews, I was constantly reminded how relatively easy it was for participants to get access to poisons and prescriptive drugs. According to Dr. X, one of the analyzers:

> We don't have enough research in the country to guide policy, legislation, anything... Checks and enforcements are needed for Pharmacy

regulations and regulations of the Poison Pesticides Board, especially for controlled substances.

It is essential to restrict access to all dangerous drugs. Education and training programs in poison awareness, labeling, and secure storage must be implemented. Persons who are known to have attempted suicide have a high suicide risk factor, and hospitals and community health centres must have a clear procedure to help them not to reattempt suicide.

Finally, socially responsible media reporting is essential to avoid copycat suicides. Yaqub, Beam and John (2017) state that:

> To encourage the responsible reporting of suicide as a public health issue, media recommendations have been developed… We find that while the journalists interviewed want to cover suicide responsibly, and as a public health issue, they often deviate from recommendations. In many cases, professional conventions and routines conflict with or hinder guideline compliance. Moreover, many journalists deliberately disregard suicide reporting guidelines because they clash with their professional values and perceived responsibility of serving the public via truth-telling and full disclosure of information. (p. 1)

More training must be provided to all levels of journalists as they report on sensitive suicide issues, particularly to ensure they do not sensationalize nor display detailed graphic pictures of the incident.

Other Concluding Observations

The research has been on Indo-Guyanese suicides. Working with the suicide participants has enabled me to share in the lives of some very special persons. I may not be of the same ethnicity nor have the same religious beliefs as some of them, but I was allowed a space by the participants to reflect on how important it is to make oneself available to be used to usher in shalom, and shalom is possible with the introduction of the transformational interventions. I followed up my research with a regional tour of some shelters housing a number of abused persons, and held seminars and counselling sessions while raising awareness of my findings and seeking ways to mitigate suicides.

I am grateful to Dr. X. who helped me to arrange some seminars in the regions with the highest suicidality which formed the basis of my research.

Having spent many years developing organizations in the UK, I strongly believe businesses should be about the triple bottom line concept. The accounting reporting framework should not only be based on financials but on social and environmental factors. Businesses should be able to focus on the needs of their communities and how they can help people to make right life choices. Now that I have been privileged to share in the pain of the research participants, I can now more fully recognize how my organization Ephrathah embraces an important vision and purpose. Ephrathah's aim is to help those who are hurting by, for example, providing psychosocial counselling through its 'Building People' arm. The counselling and personal development programs which Ephrathah provides are essential to support those who are experiencing suicide ideation or triggers leading to it. Finally, Ephrathah is set up to serve all ethnicities in Guyana and to collaborate with other like-minded agencies for this purpose.

Summary

This chapter concludes the research by providing a summary of the principles learnt and by highlighting areas for future research. I discussed some events that I was involved in following the research. I also reflected on the role of my organization in Guyana and proffered some concluding observations.

REFERENCE LIST

Barnová, S. and Gabrhelová, G. (2017). Resilience in schools. Retrieved from https://www.researchgate.net/profile/Silvia_Barnova/publication/320490507_Resilience_in_Schools/links/59e87865a6fdccfe7f8ca452/Resilience-in-Schools.pdf

Fleischmann, A., Bertolote, J. M., Wasserman, D., De Leo, D., Bolhari, J., Botega, N. J., De Silva, D., Phillips, M., Vijayakumar, L., Varnik, A., Schlebusch, L. and Thanh, H. T. T. (2008). Effectiveness of brief intervention and contact for suicide attempters: a randomized controlled trial in five countries. *Bulletin of the World Health Organization*, 86(9), 703–709.

Peltz, T. (2017). Suicide Prevention: Do San Francisco AFSP Community Walks Reduce Hopelessness?. *Master's Projects.* 554. Retrieved from http://scholarworks.sjsu.edu/cgi/viewcontent.cgi?article=1554&context=etd_projects

Pompili, M., Serafini, G., Innamorati, M., Dominici, G., Ferracuti, S., Kotzalidis, G. D., Serra, G., Girardi, P., Janiri, L., Tatarelli, R., Sher, L. and Lester, D. (2010). Suicidal behavior and alcohol abuse. *International Journal of Environmental Research and Public Health,* 7(4), 1392–1431.

Prinstein, M. J. (2008). Introduction to the special section on suicide and nonsuicidal self-injury: A review of unique challenges and important directions for self-injury science. *Journal of Consulting and Clinical Psychology,* 76(1), 1.

Shneidman, E. S. (1993). Commentary: Suicide as Psychache. *The Journal of Nervous and Mental disease,* 181(3), 145–147.

Van Orden, K. A., Witte, T. K., Cukrowicz, K. C., Braithwaite, S. R., Selby, E. A. and Joiner Jr, T. E. (2010). The interpersonal theory of suicide. *Psychological Review,* 117(2), 575.

Yaqub, M. M., Beam, R. A. and John, S. L. (2017). 'We report the world as it is, not as we want it to be': Journalists' negotiation of professional practices and responsibilities when reporting on suicide. *Journalism.* Retrieved from http://journals.sagepub.com/doi/abs/10.1177/1464884917731957

VITA

Dr Jo-Ann Rowland is the Director and Founder of the Homeless Resource Centre in London, which was set up in January 2001. She is also the founder and CEO of EPHRATHAH Multipurpose Resource Centre which was set up in March 2015 in Guyana. She is also the CEO and founder of Goldoptions Counselling and Lifecoaching Services. Additionally, Jo-Ann is an Educator and Accountant. She has been involved in numerous international mission trips including a trip to South Africa where she has worked with the Xhosa people.

Effect of the research on EPHRATHAH: Multipurpose Resource Centre

Building People – EPHRATHAH will work with relevant agencies including NGOs and community leaders across the affected regions to help to mitigate the Indo-Guyanese suicide phenomenon. Professional counselling will be available for suicide attempters and family-member survivors. Training will be available for key personnel such as first responders, and health care support staff. Personal development programs will be provided to suicide attempters and family-member survivors as part of the intervention strategy following on from the diffusion of findings. The aim of this strategy is to empower individuals to understand and know who they are and how they can overcome hopelessness and psychache.

Building Faith – Shalom needs to be established in Guyana. The intervention strategies will include supporting Church leadership to provide necessary care and comfort to suicide attempters, family-member survivors and the communities affected by suicide. There will also be an outreach to work with Hindu temple leadership in the regions affected by suicide.

Printed in May 2019
by Rotomail Italia S.p.A., Vignate (MI) - Italy